Springer-Verlag

Geschäftsbibliothek - Heidelberg

Titel: Alf Breig, Skull Traction and Cervical Cord Injury

Aufl.-Aufst.: 1. Auflage

Drucker: Appl, Wemding

Buchbinder: Appl, Wemding

Auflage: 700 Ex. Bindequote: 700 Ex.

Schutzkarton/Schuber: ---

Satzart: Filmsatz/Offset

Filme vorhanden: ja

Reproabzüge vorhanden: nein

Preis: DM 78,--

Fertiggestellt: 17.2.1989

Sonderdrucke: nein

Bemerkungen: nein

Berichtigungszettel: nein

Hersteller: I. Oppelt Datum: 31.3.1989

Alf Breig

Skull Traction and Cervical Cord Injury

A New Approach to Improved Rehabilitation

In Collaboration with
John R. Silver and Michel Renard

With 31 Figures and 11 Tables

Springer-Verlag
Berlin Heidelberg New York
London Paris Tokyo

Alf Breig, M. D., Ph. D.
formerly Professor of Neurosurgery
Karolinska Hospital, Stockholm, Sweden
Norrtullsgatan 4, S-82600 Söderhamn

In Collaboration with:

John R. Silver, M. B., B. S., F. R. C. P.
(Edinburgh and London), Consultant in Spinal Injuries,
National Spinal Injuries Centre, Stoke Mandeville Hospital,
Aylesbury, Buckinghamshire, England

Michel Renard, M. D.
Neurochirurgien des Hôpitaux; Professor and Chairman,
Department of Neuroanatomy, Faculty of Medicine,
University of Nancy, Nancy, France

ISBN 978-3-540-50414-6 ISBN 978-3-662-22410-6 (eBook)
DOI 10.1007/978-3-662-22410-6

Library of Congress Cataloging-in-Publication Data. Breig, Alf, 1910- . Skull traction and cervical cord injury: a new approach to improved rehabilitation / Alf Breig in collaboration with John R. Silver and Michel Renard. p. cm. Bibliography: p.
1. Spinal cord-Wounds and injuries-Treatment.
2. Skull-Traction. 3. Vertebrae, Cervical-Wounds and injuries-Treatment. 4. Vertebrae, Cervical-Traction. I. Silver, John R. (John Russell) II. Renard, Michel, 1932- . III. Title. [DNLM: 1. Cervical Vertebrae-injuries. 2. Spinal Cord Injuries-rehabilitation. 3. Spinal Cord Injuries-therapy. 4. Traction. WL 400 B835s] RD594.3.B74 1989
617'.482044-dc 19 DNLM/DLC for Library of Congress 88-38266

Originally published by Springer-Verlag Berlin Heidelberg New York in 1989.

2121/3140-543210 - Printed on acid-free paper

To my wife Elisabeth
who as an experienced surgical nurse has for several decades believed in the validity of the concept presented here and has given me her constant moral support

Preface

In this book on the optimal treatment of the injured spinal cord we present the reasons why we consider it necessary to handle traumatized medullary tissue in accordance with the classical biological principles of wound healing in general, namely by long-term, tension-free immobilization of the spinal cord. Today, such immobilization for this purpose can only be achieved by surgical securement of slight dorsiflexion of the cervical spine.

Traumatically compressed medullary tissue is invariably attenuated and weakened. On application of skull traction, the weakened section of the compressed cervical cord is the part that is most overstretched. This inevitably results in increased neurological deficit. On scrutiny of the clinical records of 100 tetraplegic patients treated by skull traction at the National Spinal Injuries Centre at the Stoke Mandeville Hospital, Aylesbury, England, from 1971 to 1982, we found that therapeutic skull traction had been followed by an immediate increase in neurological deficit in 12% of the patients - a relatively high figure for the type of case in which beneficial effects of traction were habitually anticipated. Moreover, in studies on cadavers, artificial defects in fresh human cervical cord in situ showed typical deformation following application of traction, confirming the basic deleterious effects of therapeutic skull traction on the injured cervical cord. On the basis of these and other observations, it must be concluded that the use of skull traction should be dropped from the treatment of spinal cord injury and replaced by immobilization of the spinal cord in its relaxed state.

The present investigations are based on our previous observations on the biomechanics of the central nervous system, published in 1960, which attracted widespread attention. It was demonstrated that, when the spinal canal shortens during dorsiflexion of the spine, the tissue of the cord is telescoped, i.e. viscously relaxed, thus producing folds. These folds are drawn out again, and the medullary tissue is elastically stretched when the spinal canal lengthens during spinal ventroflexion (6-8 cm longer in maximum ventroflexion then in maximum dorsiflexion). Shortly after our report on the physiological slackening of the shortened spinal cord, the *Medical World News* (9 September 1960) foresaw "a fundamental change in the treatment of spinal lesions" by exploitation of cord relaxation through dorsiflexion of the cervical spine.

It took a number of years, however, before the beneficial effects of cord relaxation could be confirmed in a sufficiently large number of patients with medullary lesions to allow introduction of this measure into therapy. Subsequently, cord relaxation led in a score of such patients to a remarkably high rate of restoration of neurological functions, indicating that a relatively large number of nerve fibres in spinal pathways can escape permanent damage through compression, and that relaxation is indeed an effective measure for restoration of dormant conductivity of axially oriented nerve fibres in undamaged medullary pathways.

Other researchers - for example, M. R. Dimitrijevic, Houston, and P. D. Wall, London - have arrived at similar conclusions from their respective points of departure, namely that the great majority of spinal cord lesions are in fact partial. Wall therefore proposes that treatment should be aimed at reorganizing and controlling existing connections rather than at curing the original lesion.

For these reasons, all rehabilitation experts should today be made familiar with the observation that in a significant number of patients who are disabled as a result of compressive spinal cord injury, the cord still possesses a certain degree of conductivity that can be suppressed by traction and enhanced by relaxation.

These facts prove the erroneousness of the conventional view that compressive cord injury invariably implies a death-blow to all cord conductivity. In the light of the insight presented here - namely that the effects of even slight stretching of injured medullary tissue can falsely indicate irreversible damage, whereas in reality its conductivity is only suppressed - none of the victims of traumatic cord compression can be considered to have regained his or her optimal neurological functions even after extensive and successful physiotherapy. This goal is not attained until the injured spinal cord has been relaxed by surgically secured telescoping and shortening, and the consequent reorganization of the medullary tissue has allowed the dormant neurological functions to be restored.

We feel it is extremely important to draw general attention to our simple surgical remedy of fixing the neck in barely noticeable dorsiflexion (cervicolordodesis), and in this book we describe in detail the various aspects and implications of this method. We consider it a social obligation to victims of spinal cord injury to bring these therapeutic possibilities to the knowledge of both chronically disabled persons and rehabilitation specialists.

Readers interested in more details of the principles of stress in soft nervous tissue and pathways of the pons-cord tract are referred to the author's handbook *Adverse Tension in the Central Nervous System* (Almquist and Wiksell, Stockholm, 1978).

The plan of this work matured in 1985 during a long stay by the author at the University of Gothenburg as guest of Prof. Lars Sullivan (Head of the Spinal Injuries Unit, Sahlgren Hospital) and

Prof. Annica Dahlström (Head of the Department of Neurobiology). We would like gratefully to thank both these colleagues for generously providing research facilities.

We are indebted to the Swedish insurance company Folksam, Stockholm, for financial support of the epidemiological studies in the United Kingdom.

We also wish to extend our gratitude to Mrs. Maud Marsden, Uppsala, for her expert linguistic revision of the manuscript.

Finally, we express our sincere thanks to Dr. Ute Heilmann, our Editor at Springer-Verlag, Heidelberg, for her interest and her invaluable help in achieving the present format of this book, and to acknowledge the valuable contribution of Ms. Kersti Wagstaff of the Springer-Verlag staff, who reviewed the manuscript.

Söderhamn, January 1989 A. Breig

Contents

Part I
Aggravation by Therapeutic Skull Traction of Cervical Cord Injury

1 Compressive Cervical Cord Injury and Therapeutic Skull Traction

1.1 Introduction

The term "traction" - qualified by "skull", "cervical", "spinal" and "halopelvic" - is used throughout this volume to describe traction exerted on the cervical column and thereby on the cervical spinal cord.

A knowledge of the properties of medullary tissue and the biomechanics of the spinal cord is essential for successful treatment of patients with cord injury and hence to the understanding of the topic of this book. Since, in connection with tetraplegia, interest is focused mainly on the cervical cord, prominent place is given to the description of pathological and physiological forces acting on (and in) this section of the spinal cord. Specific characteristics are described in detail in the appropriate sections; a brief outline here will serve as preliminary background information.

Lengthening of the cervical canal upon ventroflexion of the neck stretches the medullary tissue elastically; upon dorsiflexion of the cervical spine the medullary tissue relaxes into loose, undulating folds (Fig. 1). The dual nature of the cord plasma, extending upon elastic stretching and contracting upon viscous relaxation, allows immediate adaptation of the cord to the length of the spinal canal (range 6-8 cm). As recent measurements have shown [36], the conductivity of the cord for evoked potentials is not affected by changes in the length and shape of the cord or in the axis cylinders.

As shown in Fig. 2, the rhombic network of connective tissue fibres in the pial mesh enables the pia mater (and hence the cord) to respond automatically to ventroflexion and dorsiflexion of the spine by elongation and shortening, respectively. Stretching of the cervical cord reduces its cross-section, which expands again upon shortening of the cervical canal.

Figure 3 a demonstrates the visco-elasticity of medullary pulp, which retracts to its former state upon the release of tension (e.g. after termination of skull traction), provided that it has not been stretched beyond the limits of its intrinsic elasticity. In the latter case, increasing attenuation and eventual rupture result.

Traumatic compression of the cervical cord causes overstretching at the level of the compressing body; an axially oriented, oval-shaped stress field results, with maximum thinning and weakening of the cord at the centre of compression. Transverse medullary rupture can occur at this site of maximum attenuation (Figs. 3 b, c, 4, 5).

The ends of nerve fibres which have been ruptured by a transverse medullary wound retract elastically and coil up into balls. Long-term tension-free surgical

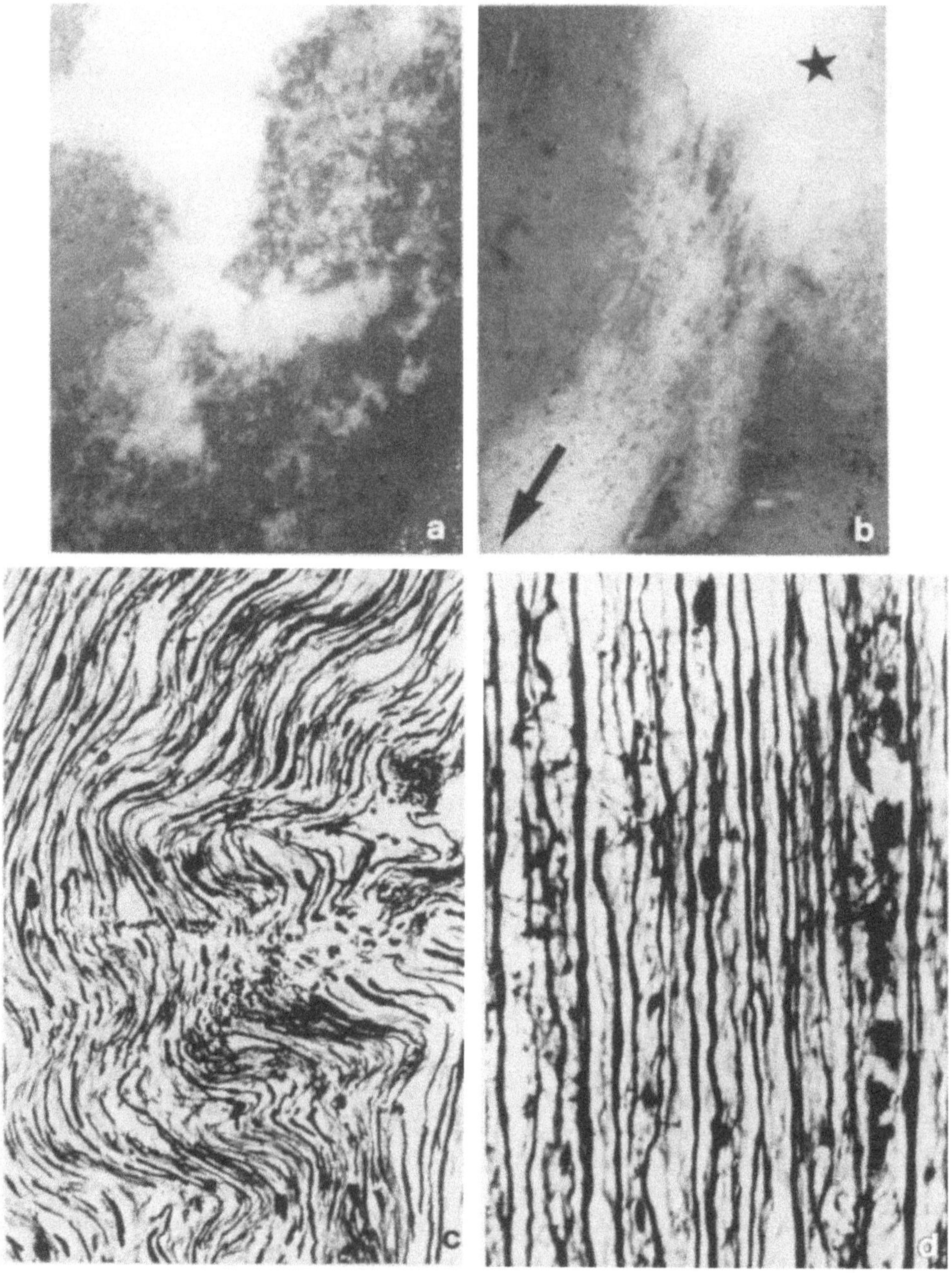

Fig. 1 a–d. Effects of viscous relaxation and elastic stretching of **a, b** disintegrated tissue and **c, d** organized medullary tissue. **a** A loose, viscous lump of plasma suspended in saline with coiled-up marginal particles. **b** Elastically stretched medullary pulp (between *star* and *arrow*). **c** Viscously relaxed and folded (cervical) medullary tissue during spinal dorsiflexion, formaldehyde-fixed in situ. **d** Elastically stretched cervical medullary tissue during spinal ventroflexion, formaldehyde-fixed in situ

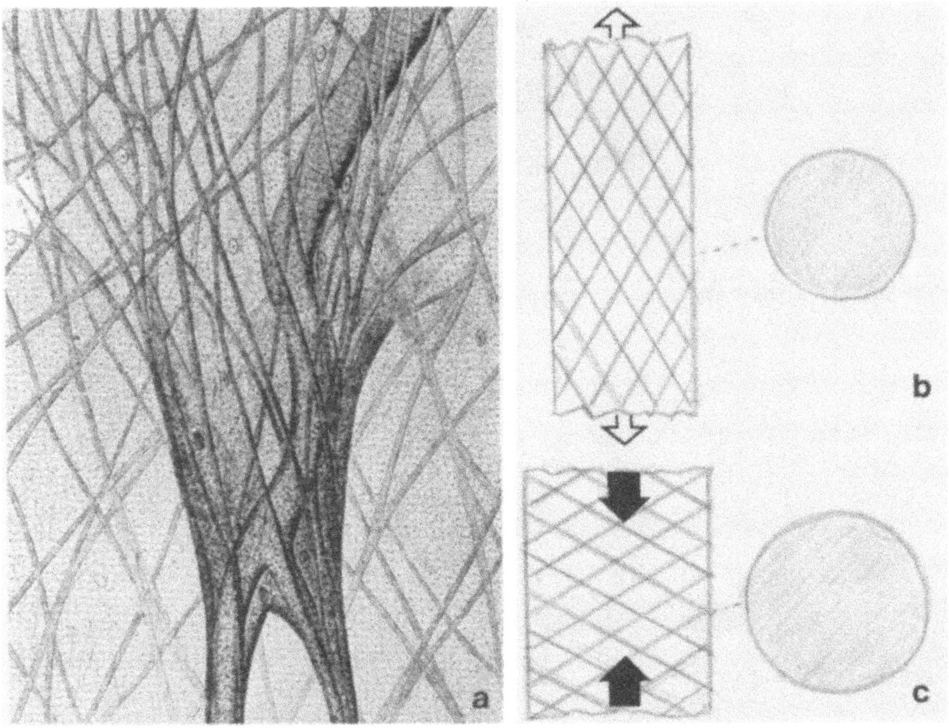

Fig. 2 a–c. Mechanism of shortening and lengthening of the pial mesh for automatic adaptation of the length of the spinal cord to the canal length. **a** Rhombic network of connective tissue fibres in canine intima piae spinalis [6]. As shown in Fig. 21, p. 56 [6], there is an identical system of rhomboidally intersecting stiff fibres in man; however, since the arrangement of these fibres happened to be more prominent in the available picture of the canine pia mater, the latter was chosen for demonstration. **b** On lengthening of the spinal canal/cord the mesh fibres intersect at acute angles. The *grey circle* shows the cross-section of the cord reduced by constriction on ventroflexion of the spine. **c** On shortening of the spinal canal/cord, the mesh fibres intersect at obtuse angles. The *grey circle* shows the cross-section of the cord enlarged on dorsiflexion of the spine. *Note:* The instantaneous arrest of cord elongation on maximal lengthening of the spinal canal is caused when undulating, vertically oriented connective tissue fibres anteriorly, laterally and posteriorly in the pial mesh are pulled taut

securement which holds the wound surfaces together enables nerve sprouts to bridge the former gap (Fig. 6).

1.2 New Insight into Deleterious Intramedullary Effects of Traction

Our suspicion that therapeutic traction on the cervical spine could inflict neurological deficit gained strong support when a follow-up X ray in a young tetraplegic patient showed that his cervical canal – compared with a film of it taken before traction – had lengthened by 10 mm during the period of skull traction.

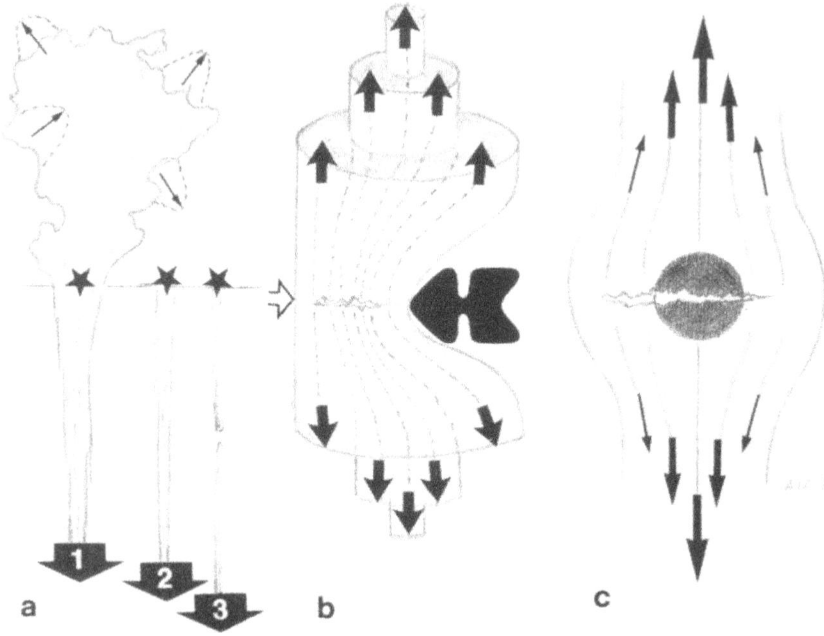

Fig. 3a–c. Legend see p. 7

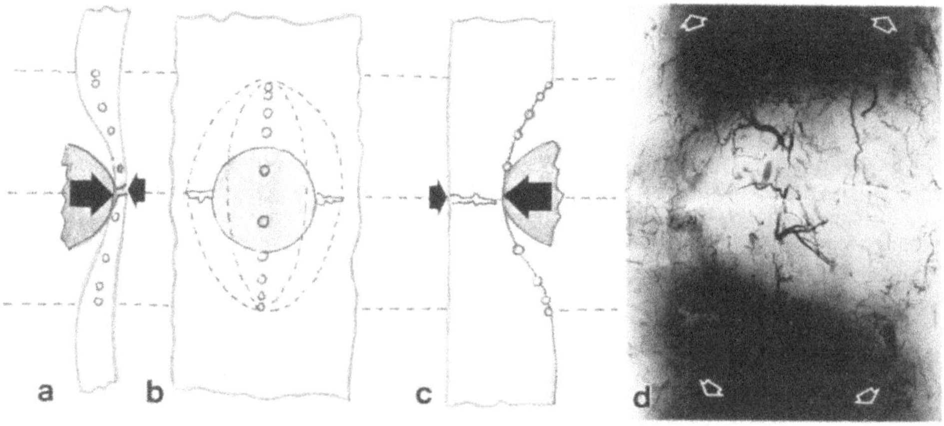

Fig. 4a–d. Range of local overstretching of medullary tissue in compression of the cervical cord. **a–c** At the centre of compression of the cord, the distances between initially equidistant markers *(small circles)* in medullary tissue are maximal, whilst the distances decrease towards the margins of the oval stress field **(b)**. **d** Microangiograph of cervical cord compressed in situ in a fresh human cadaver. From a zone of weak contrast, where the cord is thinned and weakened, most of the contrast medium is squeezed cranially and caudally by the compressing body. A transverse rupture is visible as a narrow translucent strip. At higher magnification numerous retracted and coiled-up vessels and small haemorrhages are discernible

◁ **Fig. 3a–c.** Visco-elastic properties of medullary pulp involved in normal changes in the shape and tension of the spinal cord and in its pathodynamic deformations through traumatic compression. **a** Reaction of isolated medullary pulp to micromanipulatory distraction. Non-confined pulp is viscous and deformable *(small arrows);* after release of traction equivalent to physiological stretching *(wide arrow 1),* the pulp retracts elastically to its former shapelessness. Pulp stretched beyond elastic tension becomes increasingly thinner until it finally ruptures *(wide arrows 2, 3).* **b** Propulsion profile of medullary tissue within cord cylinder in spinal cord compression. Elongation (stretching) of nerve fibres with concomitant flow of semiliquid plasma, increasing from the marginal zone to the medial and central zones. **c** Effects of compressive propulsion of medullary tissue on the shape and coherence of spinal cord (after [7]). The cord is broadened and thinned at the level of the compressing body *(black circle);* there is a transverse medullary rupture at the level of maximum stretching and thinning of the spinal cord (cf. Figs. 4, 7, 10, 12)

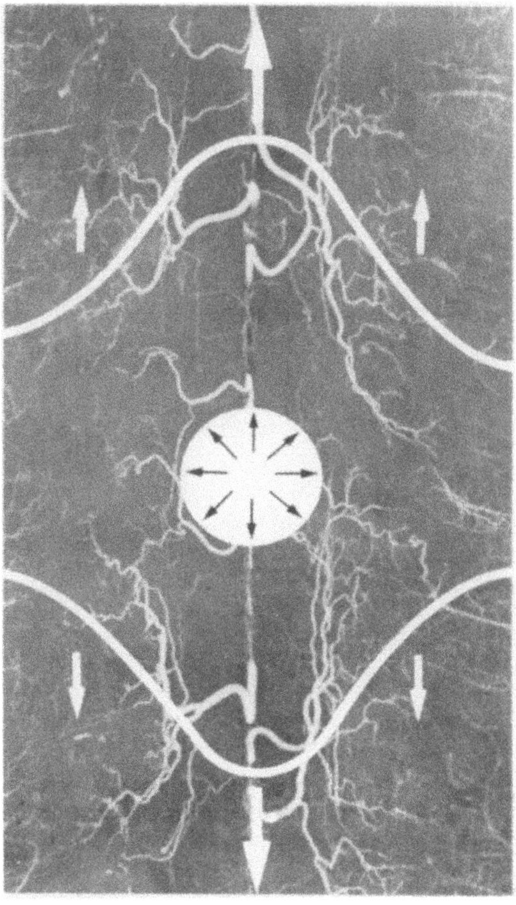

Fig. 5. Photomontage of a mid-coronal angiogram (taken from a cadaver) indicating the shape of displacement of medullary tissue during compression. The *white circle* indicates the compressing body; the other markings indicate the direction of forces. As biomechanical experiments have revealed, stretching of spinal cord tissue on compression is most marked at its centre (cf. Fig. 3): Central, axially oriented small blood vessels are therefore exposed to greater deleterious overstretching than elements in the cord periphery. (Illustration from [65])

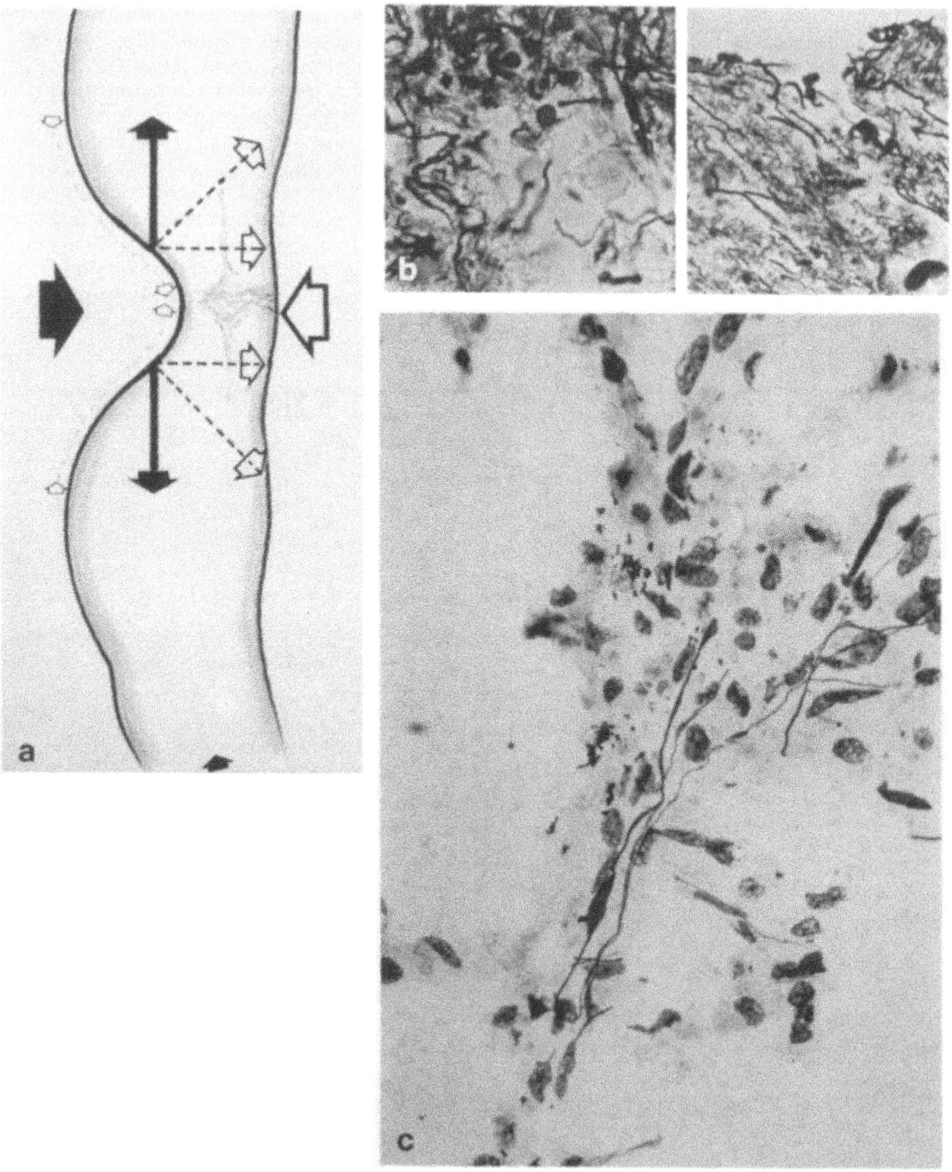

Fig. 6a–c. Experimentally produced destruction and repair in the spinal cord. **a** Diagram of reactive forces acting in a compressed cervical cord. *Long black arrows* indicate forces distracting medullary tissue to such an extent as to cause it to rupture transversely (rupture indicated by *faint lines*). *Broad arrows* indicate level of cord compression. **b** Torn medullary tissue bordering cranially and caudally on a transverse gap in deleteriously compressed cadaveric spinal cord. Numerous ruptured nerve fibres are coiled up elastically to form retraction balls. **c** Continuous nerve sprouts bridging the gap of a former hemisection cleft in canine lumbar spinal cord after surgically secured long-term, close and tension-free apposition of intramedullary wound surfaces. (From [18])

We later established by anatomical investigations that such elongation is due to the yielding of intervertebral discs and gaping of the spaces of the intervertebral joints. In the case of this patient, traction on the cervical spine was replaced by a novel measure, one which proved effective beyond expectation: his neurological symptoms regressed impressively and quickly within a few weeks as soon as his cervical spine had been immobilized in surgically secured dorsiflexion. The cervical canal was thereby shortened and the cervical spinal cord accordingly relaxed.

Case History

An 18-year-old who had sustained a diving injury presented with compression of the body of C-5 and fracture and dislocation of the left lower articular facet. Immediately after admission (Karolinska Hospital, Stockholm) 5 kg cervical traction was applied. Most neurological functions below C-5 were extinct; he was able only to lift his shoulders and abduct his upper arms slightly.

Eleven days after the injury the patient was referred to another unit, where he was submitted to the new regime: traction was immediately discontinued, and the cervical spine was dorsiflexed over a round bolster; maintenance of dorsiflexion and cord relaxation was secured by Crutchfield tongs anchored in the frontal bones and loaded with 500 g.

Twenty-four hours after spinal cord relaxation the patient regained sensibility to touch above the nipple level. Two days later the area of normal sensation extended to 5–6 cm below the nipple level. A week later, normal sensibility to light touch with cotton wool was restored in both legs and sacral dermatomes. Fourteen days after cord relaxation catheterization and bladder training could be discontinued; the range of movements in the left arm and leg had increased. Two months after admission cervical cord relaxation was made permanent by surgical fixation of the cervical spine in slight dorsiflexion (cervicolordodesis). Two weeks later spasticity in the legs diminished. The patient was able to walk short distances between bars with the aid of a splint on the right knee and a crutch-handled stick. Two years later he was largely rehabilitated, with no disabling symptoms other than a right-sided limp and slightly impaired functions of the right hand.

In this "pilot" patient – the first to be treated by spinal cord relaxation – traction had been applied on the basis of the conventional idea that reduction of bone displacement and stabilization of the cervical spine should have a favourable effect on neurological symptoms. When these symptoms remained unchanged, however, we recalled our former measurement of biomechanical changes in the shape and tension of the spinal cord in various positions of the spine [6] and began to suspect that traction might entail hitherto unconsidered dangers to the spinal cord. We therefore discontinued traction. The patient's parents opposed this unorthodox decision but were soon pleased with the results. These deliberations provided the first incentive for an investigation into the influence of the stretching of injured cervical cord on its conductivity.

To shed light on the suspected adverse influence of elastic stretching of traumatically compressed cervical cord on its conductive capacities, we began experimental analyses of the distorting effects of in situ compression of cervical cord on its constituent parts. This provided fundamental information; the distribution within cervical cord tissue of the reactive intramedullary forces generated by its compression could be mapped out, together with the deforming effects of these forces on nervous elements [7]. It was established that a prominent feature of cord compression is thinning and weakening of nerve fibres in spinal pathways, particularly axially oriented ones. From this finding it seems likely that it is the fragility of compressed (but, as clinical observations indicate, quite often surviving) nerve fibres [13, 56, 57] and their vulnerability to overstretching and possible ultimate rupturing that accounts for the deleterious effects of therapeutic skull traction and the ensuing neurological deficit.

The results of modern research into the significance of intramedullary mechanical stress in spinal cord injury have not yet been acknowledged even in recently published textbooks on the principles of spinal injury rehabilitation. This omission is apparent from the statement by an eminent rehabilitation expert on sequelae of spinal cord injury that "regardless of the nature of the bony injury, the effects on the spinal parenchyma are the same" [4]. Fortunately, a further conclusion does not hold true any more than this one, namely, that these effects ultimately result in necrosis [3, 4]. In a renewed critical discussion of this subject it has only lately been established that the great majority of spinal cord lesions are in fact partial [28]. It is true that current rehabilitation methods (e.g. immobilization of damaged spine, frequent turning and bladder training) have improved the quality of life of numerous patients with sequelae of cervical cord injury [3, 38]. However, observations are now emerging that traction can aggravate the intrinsic damage to the injured cervical cord by overstretching axially oriented nerve fibres and blood vessels in spinal pathways [7, 20, 27, 40, 55].

Such observations make it likely that replacement of traction by other stabilizing methods will in the future increase the rate of neurological improvements. On the basis of the biomechanical observations on the harmful effects of skull traction presented here, it would seem advisable, in the interest of victims of spinal cord injury, to accelerate the development of alternative orthopaedic methods for reduction of vertebral fractures and/or dislocations that would minimize unavoidable tractive forces on the cord [5, 7, 44, 54]. (In this connection, consideration will be given to the still unsolved problem of reposition of interlocked facets [58].)

1.3 Questionable Scientific Basis for Traction

It has long been known that in patients who have fractures and/or dislocations of vertebrae in association with a compressive cervical spinal cord injury, traction on the cervical spine is often successful in reducing the fractures or dislocations. For this reason, in cases of suspected cervical cord injury in accident victims many therapists today recommend traction on the cervical spine already at the scene of the injury in order to counteract compression of the cervical cord as soon as possible. As will be shown below, the present widespread assumption that traction on the cervical spine is an adequate means of protecting damaged cervical cord from further injury is not supported by any well-established mechanical or morphological facts; ill-considered recommendation of skull traction reflects the traditional disregard of potential harmful effects on the traumatically compressed cervical spinal cord.

Traction on the cervical spine can, it is true, successfully reduce or even remove pressure of dislocated bone on the cervical cord. However, since the latter is firmly anchored, cranially at the brain stem and caudally ultimately at the points of exit of the lumbosacral nerve roots, and since the spinal canal is always elongated by skull traction, this kind of traction will invariably expose the injured cervical cord to stretching [7, 25, 27, 41, 45, 54, 63].

Recent experiments have revealed that traumatically compressed cord tissue is highly susceptible to passive stretching [7]. As will be shown, traction on the cervical spine can therefore aggravate a lesion within the cervical cord of an injured person, thereby causing a considerable deterioration of his or her neurological condition. For this reason, arbitrary initiation of cervical traction without awareness of possible injury to the cervical cord, ligaments and intervertebral discs must be considered dangerous and - on the basis of the findings of the present analysis - should definitely be avoided [29, 41]. As is evident from the biomechanical measurements reported below, after a spinal injury the damaged and sensitized cervical cord must, on the contrary, be protected from adverse stretching [64]. For recently established biological reasons [7, 20], instant total immobilization of the cervical spine in the erect or - if there are no contraindications (e.g. prolapsed disc) - slightly dorsiflexed position must therefore be given high priority.

To our knowledge, no investigations into the effects of skull traction have yet been carried out. Even workers engaged in fields related directly to spinal trauma have seldom taken active interest in the way in which this widely used therapeutic procedure acts [38].

The urgent need to investigate the effects of therapeutical cervical traction has been made especially evident by the discovery that critical compression of the spinal cord invariably results in transverse rupturing [7, 61] (Fig. 7). Following research into this subject [8] it can now be easily and clearly demonstrated in experiments in situ in the rat [32] and in the fresh human cadaver [7] that the surfaces of a cervical intramedullary wound (reproducible by a transverse incision into the cervical cord) are drawn apart whenever traction (exceeding 2 kg, in the human case) is applied to the cervical spine. The consequences of this startling observation, of course, flatly contradict the previously unquestioned conventional wisdom regarding usefulness of cervical traction.

Numerous works on this issue in recent years [9, 10, 13, 15] show rehabilitation experts still to be defending themselves against the notion that cervical traction is potentially harmful. The unwillingness to entertain this view is evident in a review published by an international journal in which a critic recommended the reader to feel sceptical towards the warning about dangers of using conventionally loaded skull traction [62]. However, as the present report thoroughly documents, transverse rupturing is an unavoidable occurence at the moment of critical compression of the cervical cord; this can no longer be doubted today, even if the acceptance of this fact means a troublesome reorientation on the part of many therapists and scientific experts.

1.3.1 Anatomical Observations on Mechanical Effects of Traction

When deep neck structures in a fresh human cadaver are exposed from behind by neurosurgical techniques, a pull exerted on the cervical spine (with a pair of forceps anchored in the skull at the level of the external acoustic meatus) is seen to

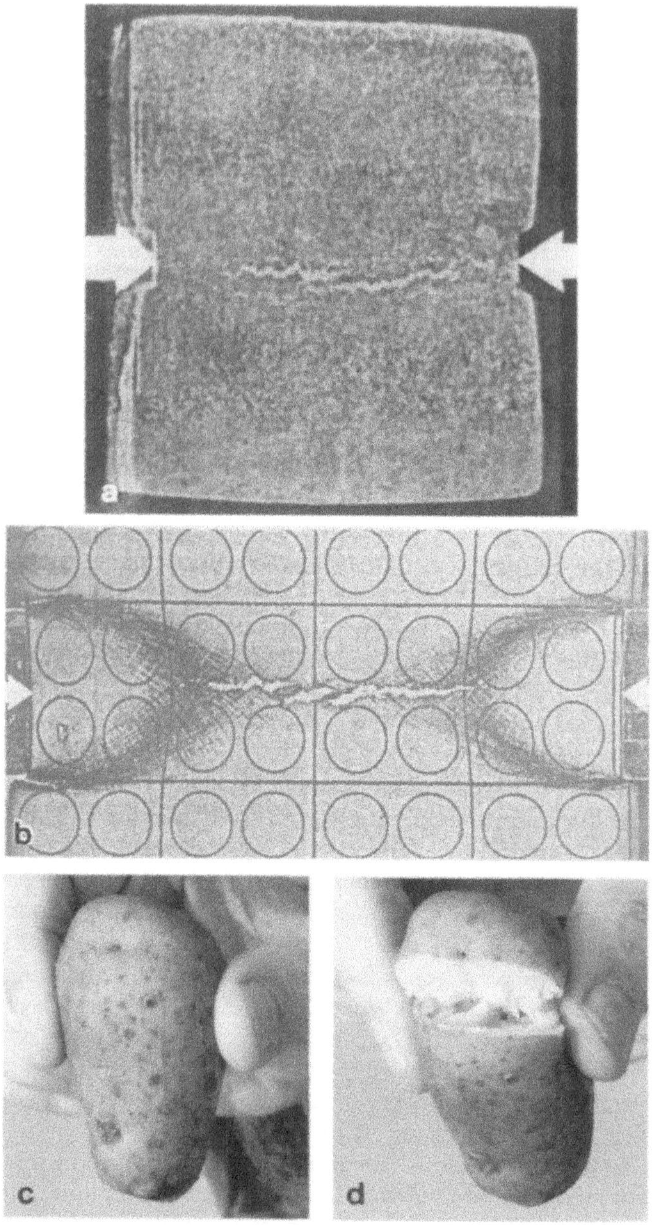

Fig. 7 a–d. Transverse crack in solid bodies regularly brought about at the level of pincer heads on compression of the bodies by critical forces. **a** Crack in a copper bar. *Arrows* indicate the points of attack of pincer heads. (Courtesy of workers at the Department of Mechanical Engineering, Royal Institute of Technology, Stockholm.) **b** Crack in a wax plate. *Arrows* indicate the points of attack of pincer heads. **c, d** Crack in a boiled potato squeezed between the thumb and the index finger

cause these structures to move towards the source of traction; the sharp edge of the light disc of the operating microscope can serve as a marker for exact measurement of the distance over which they are displaced. However, even with the naked eye cervical traction can be seen to cause changes in the shape and tension of most of the soft neck structures; for example, moderate bulging ligamenta flava are clearly straightened. After bilateral laminectomy of all cervical vertebrae, the dura mater and cervical cord are seen to be stretched moderately along their whole length, as are the dentate ligaments which attach the cervical cord to the dura mater. The upper and lower facets of the articular processes of the cervical vertebrae can clearly be observed to draw apart 1-2 mm.

The actual measurable elongation of the cervical cord is clearly produced by summation of small but constant increases in the length (i.e. in the molecular distances) of all the soft tissues and, in particular, in the length of the intervertebral discs. The latter accounts for the increase in distance between the vertebral endplates and the gaping of the articulations between the cervical vertebrae. (As would be expected, in 50-year-old patients cervical traction has been observed to cause less vertebral separation than in 20-year-olds [25].)

1.3.2 Tentative Calculation of Degree of Stretching

In the case of the pilot patient referred to on p.9, who a few days prior to his admission had sustained a cervical spinal cord injury, measurements on radiographs of the length of his cervical spine, first during cervical traction and then shortly after discontinuation of traction, showed that the cervical canal had been lengthened by 10 mm during traction with a load of 5 kg (Fig.17). None of the vertebral bodies had been damaged, except for a small vertical fissure in the anterior third of the C-5 vertebral body; all intervertebral spaces had widened equally, so that damage to discs or ligaments could be ruled out. Lengthening of the cervical canal could thus be ascribed exclusively to distension of the intervertebral discs. As an appropriate measure for elongation of the cervical canal of injured persons of average height during skull traction, it would therefore seem reasonable to add 10 mm to the length of the unloaded cervical canal; this presumes that there is no substantial damage to cervical vertebrae or discs which, through distraction, could contribute to a greater lengthening than that produced by stretching of undamaged intervertebral discs alone. (For qualifications that may justify deviation from this figure, see p.49). The elongation of the cervical canal caused by skull traction results in elastic stretching of the medullary tissue along the entire length of the cervical cord. The degree of intramedullary tension is, it is true, lower than that upon maximal ventroflexion of the cervical spine. However, as illustrated on p.6, the medullary tissue will have been thinned and weakened so much that therapeutic skull traction, even if it does not stretch the cervical cord maximally, is capable of thinning it further, thus aggravating and increasing the extent of damage to the cord.

1.3.3 Effects of Neck Postures and Traction

Table 1 gives comparative measurements and calculations that show the effects of various neck postures and methods of skull traction on the length of the cervical cord. As is evident from measurements in case 2 (row 4), the cervical cord can be stretched to a greater extent upon traction with a straight spine (assuming that 10 mm is an accurate figure for elongation of the cervical cord on traction) than upon physiological ventroflexion of the unloaded cervical spine. The former, of course, means overstretching of the cervical cord, which in itself - even without damage to medullary tissue - can reduce its conductivity. It should be the aim of epidemiological studies to ascertain how often such overstretching occurs. A biomechanical reflection may be appropriate in the present context (we shall return to this below): if skull traction with the same weight in a person with a short neck

Table 1. Effects of various postures of the cervical spine and of traction on the length of the central axis of the cervical canal/canal cord in four cadavers (cases 1-4)

	Case 1 (cm)	Case 2 (cm)	Case 3 (cm)	Case 4 (cm)
1. Length in:				
Ventroflexion[a]	13.2	12.8	13.7	11.2
Dorsiflexion[a]	10.2	10.4	10.7	8.6
Erect posture[b]	11.7	12.1	12.2	9.9
2. Elongation produced by physiological elastic stretching on changing from the erect posture to ventroflexion	1.5	0.7	1.5	1.3
3. Length attained after elastic stretching on cervical traction with cervical spine in erect posture[c]	12.7	13.1	13.2	10.9
4. Length by which elongation caused by maximum stretching on physiological ventroflexion exceeded that caused by traction on erect cervical spine[d]	0.5	−0.3[f]	0.5	0.3
5. Elongation produced by additional skull traction on maximally ventroflexed cervical spine[e]	2.5	1.7	2.5	2.3

[a] Measurements obtained from radiographs; lengths measured between tangential lines along the upper margin of the atlas and lower margin of the C-7 vertebral body.
[b] Values obtained by adding half the difference between the length of the canal in dorsiflexion and that in ventroflexion to the length in dorsi (from [6]).
[c] Values obtained by adding an average of 10 mm to the length of the cervical canal in the erect posture (cf. Fig. 17).
[d] Values obtained by subtraction of the length of the cervical canal during skull traction in the erect posture (in row 3) from its length on ventroflexion of the cervical spine (in row 1).
[e] Hypothetical values obtained by adding 10 mm (=average elongation of the cervical canal on skull traction in the erect posture with a force of approximately 4 kg) to the elongation of the cervical canal during maximum ventroflexion of the cervical spine [in (b)] (cf. Fig. 11).
[f] See p. 49.

and in another with a long neck increases the length of the cervical canal by the same amount, and if their intervertebral discs thus drawn out to an equal extent (i.e. elongation of the cord by elastic stretching is equal in both persons), it follows that the overall elastic tension in the cervical spinal cord is greater in the short-necked person than in the long-necked person and is likely to have earlier and more serious intramedullary effects. Moreover, it is logical to assume that the greater elastic intramedullary tension in short-necked patients will lead more quickly and more often to a decrease in or even disappearance of neurological function.

1.4 Beneficial Effects of Traction on Fractured or Dislocated Vertebrae

Cervical traction often succeeds in bringing together traumatically separated parts of fractured vertebrae and damaged ligaments. The reduction of fractures or dislocations is, of course, achieved by simultaneous stretching of both the anterior and posterior longitudinal ligaments; this causes them to draw towards each other, pressing on the fractured vertebrae from both the ventral and the dorsal aspects and moving them back towards or into their physiological positions.

To judge from clinical observations, the length of time needed for reduction of vertebral fragments by cervical traction can be several hours or longer. The elongation of the cervical spine that occurs during the process of such reduction is thus clearly not complete until this period has elapsed. From these observations it may probably be deduced that the force exerted on the injured cervical cord by cervical traction cannot attain its full intensity before the normal length of the cervical canal has been restored.

1.5 Historical Reasons for Delay in Documentation

Until recently relatively little work has been published on the deleterious effects of traction on traumatically compressed cervical spinal cord. One reason for this is that the biomechanics of the spinal cord and associated nerve roots and the elastic properties of most of the components of the medullary tissue were not elucidated until 1960 [6]; furthermore, the fact that the mechanical laws governing deformation of solid bodies also apply to deformation of soft spinal cord tissue was not established until 1978 [7]. Compression of the cervical cord has similar physical effects within its substance, namely thinning and weakening of its tissue, a process terminating in transverse rupturing of this tissue.

In retrospect, it is understandable that the harmful effects of cervical traction could not be recognized before the mode of action of the forces, of two different origins, was known. Moreover, these two forces come into action at two different (usually immediately successive) moments in time: (a) At the moment of cord compression, the medullary tissue in the constricted section is invariably overstretched, becoming thinned and weakened to a degree at which it is prone to rupture (see above). (b) When only thinning has occurred, and the spinal cord is elongated, either physiologically upon ventroflexion of the cervical spine or by cervical traction, the thinned and weakened section of the compressed cord invariably comes under increased tension. If the cord tissue has ruptured, the surfaces of the intramedullary wound are drawn apart upon ventroflexion of the cervical spine or cervical traction.

2 Mechanics and Biomechanics of Pons-Spinal Cord Section of Central Nervous System

In 1977, a Nobel prize winner, Rosalyn Yalow, Brooklyn, together with other participants in an interview, was asked which methods she considered might offer new opportunities for settling hitherto unsolved biological problems. She ventured the guess that it might well be mechanical methods which would open new avenues and lead to new solutions. An example which may justify this view would seem to lie in the understanding of mechanical problems inherent in spinal cord injury and their biological implications. It seems very likely that the fact that no consideration has been paid to the intriguing mechanical and biomechanical aspects of such injury has so far blocked the way to finding practicable possibilities for treating it surgically with a satisfactory outcome.

It is essential to apply sound biomechanical principles to the treatment of patients with acute spinal cord injury and to discontinue deleterious therapeutic methods which flout these principles. Even in recent publications about sequelae of spinal cord injury the biomechanics of the pons-spinal cord tissue tract is still largely disregarded. It would seem necessary to meet this deficiency by a reminder of the existence of this uniquely specialized part of the central nervous system, the functional properties of which offer essential means of automatic repair of mechanically damaged spinal cord. One of the striking properties of this tract is the capacity for viscous relaxation of the medullary tissue upon telescoping of the cord caused by dorsiflexion of the cervical spine [6, 14, 18]; this is able to promote the healing of intrinsic medullary wounds and a variety of other intrinsic pathological conditions, an ability not yet fully recognized and practically exploited.

A physiological feature of all components of spinal cord tissue is their faculty for immediate and total adaptation to the continuous changes in shape and tension of the spinal cord brought about by the normal movements of the spinal column [6, 64]. These phenomena are unparalleled in the rest of the central nervous system, for example, in the brain, diencephalon and cerebellum. The normal biomechanics of the spinal cord is deranged by - among other changes - traumatic compression of the cord; the destructive effects of the latter terminate, as shown above, in local overstretching of the axoplasm and membranes of nerve fibres in spinal pathways, resulting in thinning, weakening and ultimate tearing.

2.1 Effects of Subcritical and Critical Compression

A coherent picture has recently crystallized of the destructive intramedullary effects of traumatic compression of the cervical spinal cord and, subsequently, of the effects of physiological stretching of the cord - including its traumatized section -

when the spinal canal is lengthened, either upon ventroflexion of the cervical column or during cervical traction.

With knowledge of these effects it is possible to distinguish clearly between two well-defined degrees of compression: (a) low-grade (subcritical) compression, resulting in *thinning and weakening of the medullary tissue,* and (b) high-grade (critical) compression (for biomechanical definition, see below), which in addition to thinning and weakening leads invariably to sudden *transverse rupturing of the medullary tissue* (Fig. 8). This distinction is of importance not least in view of the different clinical significance of these two degrees: the effects of low-grade compression of the medullary tissue are to a certain extent reversible, but those of high-grade compression are always irreversible [7].

The clearly dissimilar effects of different compressive forces can be reduced to two basic mechanical events which are found to take place both in inorganic homogeneous solid bodies (HSB) and in organic bodies (e.g. the spinal cord). (For reasons given below and elsewhere [7, 8] the latter can be regarded in the same terms as HSB.)

1. Reactive tension in the spinal cord or in an HSB produced upon *subcritical compression* by pressure of pinching or clamping bodies (by definition harder than the compressed body) tends to thin them at the level of compression. In the case of the spinal cord the substance thereby displaced is pushed in opposite directions, at right angles to the level of compression cranially and caudally.
2. Reactive tension in the spinal cord or in an HSB produced by *critical compression* invariably results in a sudden transverse crack in its substance at the level of the attacking pincer heads (for mechanical evidence of reaction of the spinal cord as a solid body, see [7] and Figs. 7, 8).

The significance of this is that an increasing degree of compression will have the following consequences: Upon *shallow* encroachment of fractured and/or dislocated bone on the cord, a relatively small number of nerve fibres are thinned and weakened by cranial and caudal displacement within their sheaths. Upon *deeper* encroachment on the cord, causing more marked flattening, a larger amount of cytoplasm is sequeezed and displaced, and a larger number of nerve fibres are damaged. In the course of these events, the reactive tension within the medullary tissue inevitably attains a critical level at which the tissue suddenly ruptures transversely.

The occurrence of transverse rupturing is well documented in solid materials of varying density, at the moment when intracorporeal tension perpendicular to the transverse axis of their compression becomes critical (Fig. 7). Spinal cord tissue, because of the high water content of its constituent cell elements, also reacts as a solid body and undergoes accordingly a sudden transverse rupture under similar conditions (Figs. 8, 16). However, transverse rupture (fissure) of medullary tissue, making a superior and an inferior intramedullary wound surface, has seldom been documented to date. One probable underlying reason for this is that pathologists usually examine only transverse histological sections of injured spinal cords. Another reason may be that the detection of such a fissure with electron microscopy is impossible because of the restricted visual field.

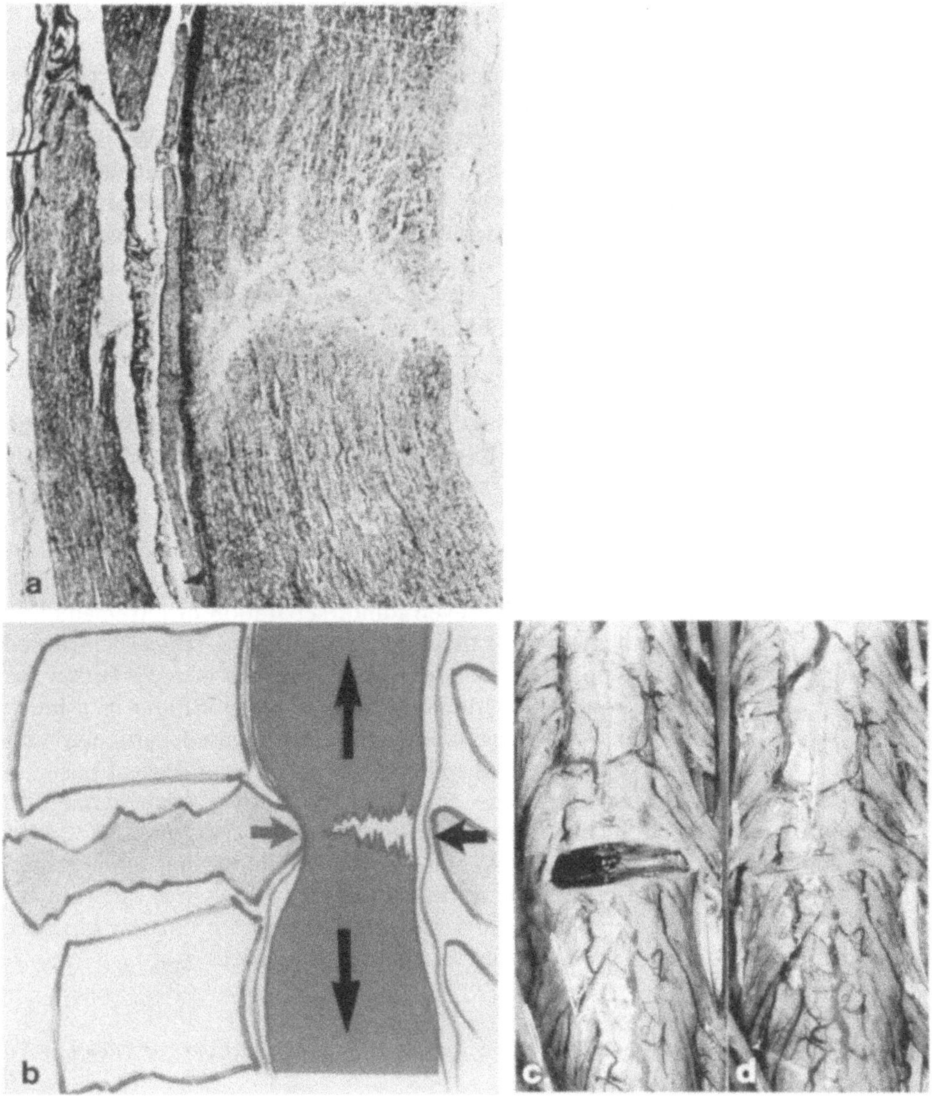

Fig. 8a–d. Transverse intramedullary rupture, a regular physical phenomenon in a severe compressive spinal cord injury. **a** Rupture (implying an intrinsic spinal cord wound with upper and lower surfaces) in a patient's cervical spinal cord (from [61]). **b** Cord rupture at the level of maximum narrowing of the cord, effected by pincer heads and cranial and caudal displacement of medullary tissue. **c, d** Transected cervical spinal cord with preserved anchorages in a fresh human cadaver, as a model of transverse cord rupture. **c** On ventroflexion and elongation of the canal, the cord sections cranial and caudal to the rupture are drawn apart. **d** On dorsiflexion and shortening of the canal, the wound surfaces are brought back into close contact (from [7])

2.2 Adverse Effects of Traction by Type of Cord Damage

As is evident from the different outcomes of compressive trauma described above, skull traction can have two different mechanical effects on damaged medullary tissue. In the case of thinned and weakened medullary tissue, traction inevitably leads to deterioration in its condition by causing continuous overstretching. In the event of rupture of the tissue, on the other hand, traction draws the intramedullary wound surfaces apart, making a considerable gap. The hypobarism created within this gap causes serum and blood to be sucked into this space. This obviously paves the way for the ingrowth of glious and possibly also connective tissue into the medullary gap, an event generally regarded as the major enemy of neurological rehabilitation – the formation of a scar is today still an insuperable barrier to return of function.

Gaping of the post-traumatic intramedullary fissure is also produced by skull traction when the cylinder of the pia has remained undamaged; to judge from a number of our earlier observations on surgically exposed cervical cord in patients shortly after a compressive injury, this often seems to be the case [7, 19]. Moreover, skull traction may cause such gaping even when the intramedullary wound surfaces do not border on the pia cylinder (for analyses, see [7]).

It is probably realistic to assume that even minor separation of intramedullary wound surfaces can effectively prevent their reunion and the healing of ruptured nerve fibres. In this connection it should be said in advance (see p. 43) that the non-physiological forces produced by therapeutic skull traction (and to a much greater extent by ventroflexion of the cervical spine) are focused particularly on thinned, weakened parts of the traumatized cervical cord. Neurological observations, such as those referred to on p. 24, that skull traction was immediately followed by loss of perception of sensory stimuli in the perineal region and sudden loss of newly restored motor functions, point to the likelihood that the impaired conductivity of the nerve fibres in the intramedullary pathways was due to overstretching of their sheaths and axoplasma, slowing down and ultimately blocking both transmission of nerve impulses and axoplasmic transport.

2.3 Properties of Cervical Cord Tissue and the Deleterious Effects of Traction

2.3.1 Visco-Elasticity of Medullary Tissue and Normal Cervical Cord Conductivity

Medullary tissue is visco-elastic, that is, it has the dual innate properties of plasticity and elasticity. Micromanipulation of a small piece of medullary tissue (suspended in saline) reveals the intriguing fact that, as long as no traction is exerted on this tissue, it can be deformed in all directions without offering the slightest resistance; however, as soon as it is stretched by application of (subdeleterious) traction, it reacts by showing a tendency to retract elastically.

It was discovered nearly three decades ago [6] that during shortening of the cervical canal, when the medullary tissue becomes relaxed and plastic, this tissue telescopes into large undulating folds (Fig. 1), and that during lengthening of the canal, owing to the firm cranial and caudal anchorages of the spinal cord, it is stretched elastically. The canal length and the cord plasticity and elasticity are indeed matched exactly in that elastic tension of the spinal cord starts just at the moment when the canal and column are about to leave the erect posture; the physiological elastic tension of the cord attains its maximum when the canal and column are lengthened maximally upon ventroflexion of the spine. A transverse incision into, for example, the cervical spinal cord shows that elastic tension of the cervical cord begins exactly when the cervical canal is about to be elongated - either by traction on or flexion of the cervical spine. This is the clue to understanding the ability of therapeutic skull traction to inflict increased neurological deficit on patients with a compressive cervical spinal cord injury.

2.3.2 Reaction of Subcritically Compressed Cervical Spinal Cord to Traction

As described above, the injurious effects of therapeutic skull traction on traumatically compressed cervical spinal cord depend on the *degree* of short-range axial overstretching to which the compressed section of the cervical cord was subjected at the moment of its traumatic compression.

In a section of cervical cord constricted by intruding bone it is mainly the axis cylinders that are flattened and narrowed, so that their cytoplasma is sequeezed out from the constricted section. Moreover, since pressure on any solid body is mechanically converted into tension within that body, it follows that both the membranes and the axoplasma of the axis cylinders are overstretched within the constricted section of the cervical cord. These mechanical events cause the considerable thinning of the cervical spinal cord along its compressed section. Because of the relatively high resistance of the spinal pia sheath (which is reinforced by coarse connective tissue fibres; see Fig. 2 and [6, 43]) to sudden horizontal widening and because of the predominantly axial course of the tissue elements in the compressed cord section, stretching and thinning of the medullary tissue take place mainly axially. The degree to which noticeable thinning of the cord is caused and the distance over which thinning occurs depend on the shape and size (surface area) of the impinging bone and on the depth and speed of its intrusion [7]. As is visible in specimens from fresh human cadavers, even relatively shallow impingement of the compressing body on the cervical cord always causes a certain number of axis cylinders and blood vessels to be overstretched, thinned and weakened. This model shows, moreover, that the greater the compression (i.e. thinning), the greater is the number of conducting elements that are endangered. Axis cylinders that have survived this stress and are perhaps only imperceptibly lengthened are extremely liable to lose their conductivity with any additional tension. This has been verified by, among others, neurological surgeons [20, 35, 42, 46] who have observed that critical tension of nerve fibres abolishes their conductivity, and that their conductivity can be restored by relaxation of the fibres, as long as they are basically undamaged. Thus, the experimentally verified pull on the cervical spinal cord exerted by skull traction and the consequent stretching of the cervical medullary tissue inevitably reduce the conductivity of still resistant nerve fibres and irreversibly damage those that cannot withstand this strain.

2.4 Neurology of Spinal Cord Overstretching

Medullary biomechanics and pathodynamics have recently opened a novel dimension in neurology. This knowledge allows demarcation of a specific group of neurological symptoms, all of them characterized by the fact that they are triggered by local distortion of the medullary tissue. Although unspecific, the pattern of this deformation of spinal cord tissue varies widely with the location, shape and size of the offending lesion. Analysis of a great number of acute and chronic clinical medullary disorders has revealed medullary distortion as the symptom-triggering factor. Knowledge of the biomechanics in question allows understanding both of the nature of the characteristic adverse effects of cervical traction and of the beneficial effects of surgically secured spinal cord relaxation.

Besides its manifold intricate morphological and physiological specializations, the spinal cord is not least a simple cord of soft tissue with certain characteristic mechanical, biomechanical and biological properties [6, 7, 31]. As such, it reacts to any pathological load placed upon it, through various indurative changes outside of or within its substance, by local overstretching. This basic phenomenon implies, of course, that any hard intra- or extramedullary change exposes axis cylinders and small blood vessels in the immediate vicinity of the pathological focus to abnormal stretching. Examples of firm bodies (changes) which bring about this effect *from within* the spinal cord are scar formation after spinal cord injury, space-occupying intramedullary tumours, haemangiomata, cysts and oedema, i.e. processes of widely different origin. Firm bodies causing local overstretching of medullary tissue *from without* include osteophytes (such as those causing cervical myelopathy), intracanalicular tumours, spinal deformity and bone fragments.

Since overstretching of nerve fibres in spinal cord pathways is invariably brought about in the same manner irrespective of the greatly varying nature of the actual changes within or outside of the spinal cord, it can be reduced either partly or completely by cervicolordodesis (CLD). After unspecific relaxation by this measure, neurological symptoms of the category in question either partially or totally regress. The favourable reaction of our pilot patient (p. 9) confirmed that even neurological symptoms after a spinal cord injury can be reduced by CLD insofar as they are caused by mechanical stress in, and not by destruction of, conducting nervous elements. This important fact was later documented clinically in a number of patients [7, 13, 20]. As CLD is capable of reducing or completely relieving sensory, motor and vegetative neurological symptoms of the above aetiology, the CLD surgeon has at his disposal a wide-range therapeutic tool. Workers who have followed the development of this biological surgery now tend to see CLD as a new, highly efficient method that can improve the neurological condition of a large number of patients with disorders characterized by focal overstretching of the medullary tissue.

2.4.1 Neurological Efficacy of Spinal Cord Relaxation

The therapeutic range of cord relaxation is clear from its beneficial neurological effects in a patient (a women aged 54) with cervical intramedullary scar formation treated several years after an automobile accident. This patient had sustained an injury to her cervical spine, with signs and symptoms of chronic hemi/tetraparesis and increasing urinary incontinence. After CLD relaxation of the cervical cord, the respective chronic motor, sensory and bladder symptoms regressed within a few weeks to a remarkable degree (witnessed by referring neurologists, Queen Square Hospital, London). However, when the CLD ribbon became worn out (which allowed the patient to bend her head forward to a slowly increasing extent), the neurological symptoms recurred to a proportional extent. After reoperation with renewed CLD slackening of the cervical cord (this time using an improved, non-stretchable ribbon), the neurological symptoms regressed to almost the same extent as after the first fixation of the cervical spine in a position of slight dorsiflexion. At the time of her death from pneumonia, the neurological improvement had lasted for 7 years. This experience confirmed beyond doubt that (a) it is stretching of the cervical cord that gives rise to neurological deficit, and that (b) relaxation of the cervical cord is the therapeutically effective factor, since it prevents the damaged cord from being stretched.

The possibility of restoring a dormant capacity for transmission of action potentials in injured cervical cord - i.e. cord under mechanical stress - by relaxation of the cord, as documented in this patient, opens exciting therapeutic perspectives. However, another goal that at present lies nearer at hand is the future prevention of the present extent of damage to freshly injured cord produced by "therapeutic" skull traction. Recurrence of the former distressing neurological deficit in the patient discussed above, when the relaxed (but scar-containing) cervical cord again came under tension by unintentional traction upon it, is almost tailor-made confirmation of the undeniable reality that cervical cord traction is invariably deleterious to injured cervical cord. These facts should convince all therapists of the danger caused to their patients by continued use of skull traction in such cases.

We are fully aware of the fact that the quality of fresh tractive damage to recently injured axis cylinders and blood vessels must necessarily differ from tractive damage to chronically deformed nerve fibres. There is certainly a vast field here for future research. Nevertheless, there cannot be any doubt that stretching of post-traumatically disabled nerve fibres is the common denominator for the disturbance of their transmission.

3 Deleterious Effects of Therapeutic Skull Traction: A Retrospective Study

3.1 Background

The transverse rupturing of medullary tissue which is a typical effect of (critical) cord compression can be demonstrated in a fresh human cadaver by making a transverse incision in, for example, the cervical spinal cord. Since the wound surfaces of a transverse cleft in the fresh cadaveric cord are invariably drawn apart through elastic stretching of the cervical cord upon lengthening of the cervical canal by skull traction, it may be concluded that in patients with spinal cord injury skull traction is bound to have similar adverse effects on medullary tissue that has been thinned and/or ruptured transversely upon compression.

In several patients whose clinical notes we have followed in recent years it has been observed that therapeutic skull traction was clearly followed by deterioration of their neurological functions.

In the following two patients treated in 1985, one in Sweden and the other in a hospital abroad, deleterious cord distension had obviously occurred during skull traction. The first patient, aged 53 years, with fracture dislocation of C-6/C-7 and interlocked facets (ILF), was initially treated with skull traction (12 kg). After reduction of the dislocation halopelvic traction was applied. The consequent stretching of the cervical spine led to marked deterioration of the patient's neurological state, with bilateral annulment of arm extension, reduced function of the biceps muscles, a sensation of "pins and needles" in both arms and abolition of sensibility in both hands [34]. The shoulder muscles also showed decreasing function, and the anal and bulbocavernosus reflexes disappeared. A renewed X-ray check revealed a pathological increase in the distance between the C-6 and C-7 vertebral bodies [30]. The traction was therefore immediately reduced to 2.5 kg. On the following morning the function of both biceps muscles had returned to normal. Bilateral surgical laminectomy was carried out thereafter (in our opinion, on a questionable indication), with no return of any of the neurological functions that had been present before the traction therapy was begun.

The second patient, treated abroad, was a 22-year-old man with a cervical spinal cord injury, about whom we were recently consulted. On admission to hospital he still had perineal sensibility and toe movements, but these functions disappeared soon after skull traction was begun.

3.1.1 Anticipated Obstacles to Clinical Confirmation

Sometimes the patient is put under traction while he is in a state of spinal shock, so that any adverse effects of this treatment are concealed and therefore usually not recorded. Moreover, in the acute state of injury any visible reduction of the range or grade of neurological functions cannot always be followed thoroughly because other events of vital importance to the patient must be attended to. It is readily understandable under these stressful circumstances that neurological changes may either escape notice or, if observed, be seen as related to various other factors. Another probable obstacle to the recognition of early adverse neurological effects of traction on the cervical cord is the occurrence of slowly increasing oedema 3-4 h after the injury, the effects of which on neurological functions can, of course, overshadow possible adverse effects of traction.

If, on the other hand, the patient shows signs of neurological improvement soon after discontinuation of skull traction (cf. case report, p.9), this is likely to be either not fully recorded or considered as a self-evident positive effect of rehabilitation measures and therefore probably not ascribed to termination of traction. Thus, many circumstances may obscure proper evaluation both of possible drawbacks connected with skull traction and of advantages to the patient when this method is used either not at all or with the precautionary measures mentioned below.

Attempts to make an objective evaluation of deleterious effects of skull traction on an injured cervical cord are hampered, moreover, by the fact that the traditionally presumed beneficial effects of this method on the healing of injured cervical vertebrae and ligaments divert any suspicion as to its possible dangerous consequences. Understandably, there is no room for neurological assessments during eager expectancy of the time when the spine is consolidated, and the patient can be seated upright and rehabilitated by the physiotherapeutic training programme tailored specifically for him and which, as is known from ample experience, will bring noticeable and vital improvement. Thus, the apparently pleasing prospects for the rehabilitated patient can ultimately prevent the observer from arriving at the doubtless shocking idea that the patient's neurological condition may have been a good deal better still if, during the acute stage of the injury, his cervical cord had not been subjected to traction and thus probably further damaged.

3.2 Analysis of Clinical Records

It was thought that more light might be shed on these questions by an epidemiological study of the effects of skull traction therapy - by scrutiny, for example, of entries in clinical records of specialized departments of hospitals in which relatively large numbers of patients had been treated with skull traction. The author obtained the opportunity to carry out such an investigation at the National Spinal Injuries Centre at the Stoke Mandeville Hospital (SMH), Aylesbury, in England. The clinical reports were examined here on 100 tetraplegic patients who had been treated by skull traction during the period 1971-1982. The present judgements concerning neurological changes are based only on patients who were treated with traction and who showed gradual improvement.

Many of the SMH clinical records contain notes about treatment begun overseas. These confirm that therapeutic traction is today a generally adopted method, and that this treatment is employed uniformly throughout the world. Moreover, it is apparent that delayed application is now universally regarded as an inexcusable omission. This adherence to a currently valid doctrine points to the likelihood that a future ban on skull traction will not readily be approved until the weighty arguments in favour of its abandonment have been generally accepted.

3.2.1 Types of Injury and Their Treatment

One-third of the cervical spinal cord injuries reviewed in this study had resulted from traffic accidents, and 23% were due to falls from a height; the remainder had occurred during sports activities (Table 2). Post-traumatic confusion was experienced in two cases: a 29-year-old patient (case 51) was "confused for first few days", and a 41-year-old patient (case 64) was "slightly confused" on admission. Injuries at the level C-5/C-6 had occurred in 26% of cases, at C-6/C-7 in 16% and at C-4/C-5 in 12%; a further 12% of patients had injuries at the level of vertebra C-5 (Table 3).

Twelve patients had ILF; as can be seen from Table 4, the majority of ILF were at vertebral levels C-5/C-6 and C-6/C-7. Table 4 also shows the weight of traction and the special supportive procedures applied in each of the 12 cases of ILF.

In 27 of the cases in this study the duration of traction was not recorded; the average duration in the remaining 73 cases was 43 days. The applied traction load ranged from 2.3 to 20.7 kg. Of the various types of traction recorded, Crutchfield tongs were the most frequently used (in 28 cases). Table 5 gives a survey of the traction treatment administered. Calipers fell out on 16 occasions, causing failure of traction.

Case 82 serves as an example of the varying therapeutic strategies practised during treatment of an injury to the cervical spine:

Table 2. Types of accident causing cervical spine injury in 100 patients at Stoke Mandeville Hospital

Type of accident	% of cases	
Road traffic	34	
Fall from a height:	23	
Indoors		10
At work		9
Outdoors		4
Diving	15	
Motor cycle	10	
Rugby	10	
Car racing	4	
Trampoline	2	
Gymnastics	2	
	100	

- Neurological signs: "fairly severe paresis affecting the arms more than the legs".
- Traction (1.8 kg) administered in slight flexion because X ray (extension view) showed opening of C-4/C-5 disc space, indicating rupture of anterior spinal ligament; duration, 4 days.
- Well-fitting collar (in Hackney Hospital); duration, 6 days.
- Traction reapplied (after transfer to SMH) but without flexion; duration, 4 weeks.
- Neurological signs: improving after 4 weeks.

Table 3. Vertebral level of spinal injuries in SMH patients

Level of spinal injury (involved vertebrae)	Frequency of fracture and/or dislocation (%)
C-5/C-6	26
C-6/C-7	16
C-4/C-5	12
C-5	12
C-3/C-4	10
C-6	5
C-4	5
C-7/T-1	3
C-7	2
C-3	1
?	6

Signs and symptoms of tetraplegia + anaesthesia modified by level and degree of cord compression.

Table 4. Frequency of interlocked facets in SMH patients and means of reduction

Interlocked facets (level)	Frequency (%)	Case no.	Weight of traction (kg)[a]	Special supportive procedures		
				Manipulation	Open reduction	Dorsiflexion reduction
C-3/C-4	1	60	20.7		+	
C-4/C-5	2	43	5.5, 13.5		+	
		65	4.6, 9.2, 3.2	+		
C-5/C-6	4	5	8.2			
		18	6.9, 3.2			+
		34	6.9, 12.8, 2.7	+		
		81	?		+	
C-6/C-7	4	11	3.6, 2.7			
		44	?		+	
		67	9.2, 2.3	+		
		85	18.5, 13.5			
C-7/T-1	54	54	9.2	+		
	12		2.3-20.7 (range)	4	4	1

[a] Converted from avoirdupois pounds.

Table 5. Traction treatment administered to 100 SMH patients

Type of traction	Frequency of application
Unspecified (probably Crutchfield tongs)	44
Crutchfield tongs	28
Cone calipers	15
Blackburn calipers	4
Gardner-Wells calipers	3
Halopelvic apparatus	2
Halter traction	2
Sugar traction	1
Collar	1

Duration of traction was not recorded in 27 cases; average duration of traction in remaining 73% of patients was 43 days. Range of applied load: 1.8–20.7 kg.

3.2.2 Deterioration of Neurological Functions Following Traction

Cervical traction was recorded as having reduced post-traumatic pain in three instances: in one patient (case 25, aged 28), pain in the neck and shoulder girdle was alleviated; another (case 28, aged 17) experienced reduction of "tight" feeling in the head and neck; and the third (case 32, aged 24) felt "more comfortable now in head traction".

Before access had been obtained to these clinical notes, it was speculated, however, that observations would probably be sparse regarding deterioration of neurological functions shortly after the application of traction. As anticipated, the records scrutinized seldom contained such references. When such deterioration was noted, however, the observer had not, understandably enough, made any suggestion as to its possible cause. Nevertheless, from the fact that he had reported it, it would certainly seem justifiable to conclude that its manifestation must have been unexpected and probably also marked. Although not expressively stated by the SMH therapists, there are indications in these notes that the bedside observations in question caused them to think of these functional impairments – because of their manifestation shortly after commencement of skull traction – as having been provoked by the traction rather than, for example, by oedema. The distribution of the neurological deficit over various parts of the body suggests that overstretching of axons must have been focused on different central points of the medullary cross-sectional area and, accordingly, on (parts of) certain spinal pathways. Deterioration of neurological functions following skull traction was noted in the records of 12 of the 100 tetraplegic patients (Table 6). In most instances neurological deficit was observed some time after commencement of traction; in one patient ascending sensory deficit was recorded as developing "during traction procedure" (i.e. immediately after installation of traction?). Since a certain length of time is required before all cervical structures are distended, and damaged cervical cord is thus stretched maximally, it is reasonable to suppose that neurological functions usually do not begin to deteriorate until some hours after the installation of traction.

Table 6. Increasing neurological deficit after commencement of skull traction

Case no.	Age (years)	Level of injury	Special features or treatment	Time after traction commenced	Entry in clinical notes
5	45	C-5/C-6		2 days	"Anal reflex less brisk."
32	24	C-5/C-6		1 day	"Loss of finger flexion of left hand."
36	52	C-3/C-4	Brown-Séquard's paralysis	Soon	"His ability to move his left leg disappeared and the acuity of sensation in his right leg became blunted."
39	40	C-3/C-4		Soon	"Motor power in the upper limbs has deteriorated and the motor power in the left lower limb has deteriorated as well."
53	59	C-4/C-6		Soon	"Apparently he flexed his elbows when he came in."
70	20	C-5/C-6		Soon	"He had feelings in his legs right after injury."
76	20	?			"During traction procedure the sensory level had localized definitely below the C-6 dermatome." (Sensory level on admission below T-2 dermatome)
79	20	C-5	C-4/C-6 posterior fusion with wires and post-operative traction		"Sensory level last normal segment R: C-4; L: C-5 (Level before traction R: C-6–C-7, L: C-7)." (Note: see discussion below)
81	27	C-5/C-6		Soon	"Later on the same day there was a question of deteriorating sensory level, and it was decided to perform a decompression of the cervical spine." (Note: no improvement following decompression)
85	57	C-6/C-7	ILF[a]	?	"Sensory level ascended to midarm."
93	32	C-4/C-5		Soon	"He had some difficulty in breathing."
95	19	C-6		1 day	"The lesion ascended and his paralysis became more severe, going as high as C-4, but it later regressed."

From Stoke Mandeville Hospital records. Entries in the clinical notes are quoted literally.
[a] ILF, Interlocked facets.

The neurological deficiencies induced occurred in various parts of the body (Table 6): reduced sensibility in the limbs/ascending sensory level in six out of the 100 patients; reduced power of muscles of upper and/or lower limbs in four; disappearing vegetative reflex in one; and increased difficulty in breathing in one.

Compression of the cervical cord in these patients had occurred at various levels, from C-3 to C-7; no findings were recorded pointing to diastasis between damaged vertebrae and thus to a mechanism of lengthening of the cervical canal other than skull traction. No notes were made regarding the shape of the patients' necks. For various reasons the radiographs could not be scrutinized.

In addition to the various neurological deficiencies recorded in Table 6, adverse effects of traction were noted in two cases: one patient (case 36) experienced episodic dysphagia, and another (case 41) suffered from a stiff jaw after insertion of the calipers into the temporalis muscles.

Table 7 summarizes the demonstrable effects of cord deformation caused by traumatic compression and exacerbated by cervical traction.

3.2.3 Improvement of Neurological Functions Following Reduction/Termination of Traction

One patient with ILF at level C-5/C-6 (case 18, Table 4) experienced a return of sensation in the upper limbs and improved wrist movements within 2 days after his neck had been moderately dorsiflexed by means of a pillow under the shoulder blades, and traction had been reduced from 6.9 to 3.2 kg. Dorsiflexion of the cervical spine under traction also proved beneficial in case 55; after 14 days the patient "had regained light touch and proprioception in his lower limbs, and a sensory level (at C-5) was no longer detectable". In both cases, neurological functions continued to improve subsequently. Another patient with ILF (at C-3/C-4) recovered sensation in arms and legs and experienced a return of posterior tract functions following surgical securement of cervical spinal dorsiflexion of the C-2 spinous process to the spinous processes of C-4/C-5.

Reappearance of neurological functions relatively soon after termination of skull traction was noted in 7% of the SMH records (Table 8). All of these notes concerned markedly improved muscle functions in the arms and legs. However, notes about such reappearances had been made only on the first one-third of the SMH patients and not on the following two-thirds (except for a single patient), and this figure of 7% is therefore probably too low. During the years in which the first one-third of the patients were admitted the neurological symptoms were described exactly and in detail; however, during the following 6-year period the records were generally shorter and rather incomplete. (The reason why more exact notes were no longer made in the latter records is unknown.) The reappearance of motor, sensory and vegetative functions is no longer surprising in the light of work carried out some years ago by workers in the United States who succeeded by means of neurophysiological methods in revealing dormant neurological functions even in a certain percentage of patients who had had long-standing neurological deficit [28].

Table 7. Breakdown of cervical cord conductivity through thinning[a] and rupturing of axis cylinders due to traumatic cord compression; increased deficit caused by cervical traction

Anatomical studies in fresh human cadavers		Clinical observations in patients with fresh transverse sectional lesions
Cervical spinal cord compression in situ	In the presence of a transverse intramedullary rupture, physiological elastic stretching of cervical medullary tissue on ventroflexion of the spine	Therapeutic cervical traction in these patients
Causes: a) (When a–p diameter reduced by 20%) stretching and thinning of axially oriented axis cylinders and blood vessels b) (When a–p diameter reduced by more than 25%) additional transverse rupture of medullary tissue (compressive intramedullary wound with cranial and caudal wound surfaces). Extent of rupturing dependent on determinable physical factors Cervical traction (3–7 kg and more) *Causes:* Increased gaping of intramedullary wound	*Causes:* Retraction of cranial and caudal wound surfaces (gaping of intramedullary wound)	*Causes:* Non-physiological lengthening of cervical spinal canal and corresponding overstretching of injured cervical cord. Any part of cervical medullary tissue that is thinned and weakened by compression is then exposed to greater elongation than neighbouring, undamaged medullary tissue (high resistance of ligaments, discs and muscles diminishes deleterious effects of traction on cervical spinal cord/medullary tissue; low resistance of these structures increases deleterious effects on cervical cord/medullary tissue). *Clinical signs following start of traction:* Diminution or abolition of still existing neurological functions during or shortly after establishment of therapeutic cervical traction[b, c]. *Clinical signs following termination of traction:* Slow and incomplete return of certain neurological functions after early termination of cervical traction, though only if overstretching of nerve fibres has not been deleterious[c].

[a] And correspondingly reduced or abolished axonal transport and action potential traffic.
[b] Possibly masked by initial deficiency of conductivity (spinal shock, oedema).
[c] Confirmed by clinical observations and objective case reports.

Return of neurological functions (Table 9) was also noted in SMH records to have occurred (a) during long-standing skull traction and (b) immediately after establishment of skull traction. The former instance may be characterized as restoration "despite skull traction" and the latter as restoration "due to skull traction".

Table 8. Reappearance of neurological functions after termination of skull traction

Case no.	Age (years)	Level of injury	Special circum-stances	Time of neurological assessment after termination of traction (days)	Entry in clinical records
7	28	C-6		2	"Definite return of normal dorsiflexion and plantar flexion of both feet."
15	29	C-4/C-5		2	"Definite movement of left toes."
16	22	C-6/C-7		5	"Regained fairly good power in both upper limbs (except in hands)."
17	15	C-5/C-6		2	"Improved muscle power to almost normal in left leg."
22	15	C-6/C-7		5	"Definite movement of left lower limb, possible movements of right lower limb, quads and adductors."
25	28	C-5/C-6	Subjec-tively worse	2	"Crutchfield tongs fell out tonight." Two days later: "Neurologically improved."
65	28	C-4/C-5		2	"Slightly getting better."

From Stoke Mandeville Hospital records. Only such functions are mentioned which, some days before their reappearance, had been expressly pointed out in the clinical records as absent. (*Note:* The cases evaluated in the present study have been arbitrarily numbered 1-100. When, in the notes following case 25, no more entries were found concerning reappearance of neurological functions (except in case 65), it was realized that the notes of patients with numbers above 29 referred to patients admitted 6 years later.)

Neurological improvement in the former (e.g. case 28) and immediately after reestablishment of skull traction in the latter (e.g. cases 38 and 98) would seem at first glance to contradict the assertion that traction has invariably deleterious effect on the cervical cord in patients with cervical cord injury. However, this seeming exception to the rule can be shown to be spurious when all (bio)mechanical circumstances bearing on the conductivity of the cervical cord are thoroughly analysed; the reasons for the seemingly exceptional neurological reactions in the patients in question are also comprehensible. It therefore remains to be shown, in the first place, that no (or only minimal) intramedullary injury had occurred in these favourably reacting patients.

In situation (a) above (case 28), the mechanism of injury to the cord is not entirely clear from retrospectively available information. An X ray taken soon after the accident showed "reduced fracture dislocation C-5/C-6". According to the clinical record, this 17-year-old "was trapped when going down a ladder" near a helicopter "that jumped and spun over" (low-speed injury?). The fact that motor ability had already improved in both his hands and legs 4-5 days after the injury makes it obvious that possible tearing of medullary tissue must have been very slight and that - like the cervical cord tissue of the patient referred to below under

Table 9. Improvement of neurological functions by tractive reduction of non-deleterious thrust on cervical cord caused by dislocated vertebral bone

Case no.	Thrust[a]	Neurological signs on admission	X ray cervical spine	Initial treatment	Duration	Effect	Relapse	Subsequent treatment	Duration	Effect on neurological functions
28	At moment of trauma by fractured, dislocated bone	Incomplete C-5 level; motor power upper limbs fairly good except in hands. Sacral sparing and anal reflex +	Fracture/dislocation C-5/C-6	Traction 6.4 kg	1 day	Fracture/dislocation reduced soon after (commencement of) traction	None	Traction 2.7 kg	40 days	After 1 week: fairly good power in both upper limbs. After 4 weeks: "Tremendous improvement of power in right leg, some power recovery in left leg, sensory recovery of bladder and urethra."
38	Slow-speed, caused by sudden dislocation of atlas 2 days after initial trauma	Incomplete quadriplegia after extension injury	Osteophyte formation from C-3 down; slight lateral shift of atlas	Stabilization by means of collar	2 days	Some recovery of movements in most muscle groups	2 days after admission: sudden difficulty in breathing, muscle power reduced, picture of complete tetraplegia; X ray showed marked lateral shift of atlas over the axis	Emergency skeletal traction with Crutchfield tongs (load not recorded)	34 days	Immediate neurological improvement: "Neurological picture now the same as it was on his admission."
98	Slow-speed, caused by redislocated vertebral bone 10 days after termination of traction	Severe head injury; no voluntary limb movements	Fracture/dislocation C-3/C-4	Traction (weight not recorded)	35 days	After 3 weeks of traction, sudden purposeful movements of legs	10 days after removal of calipers: sudden deterioration of power in both legs	Resumption of traction (load not recorded)	Not recorded	"He was put back on skull traction with marked improvement but never regained his former power."

[a] Type of thrust on cervical cord (in case no. 38, on upper cervical cord).

situation (b) - most of it had been transiently but not deleteriously overstretched. For this reason, continued skull traction, which after the X ray diagnosis was lowered to 2.7 kg, could not have done any substantial harm. It would therefore seem reasonable to describe the clinical development of this patient as "neurological restoration despite skull traction".

In situation (b) above (case 38), the atlas vertebra, as a result of its sudden lateral shift, had pressed on the corresponding section of the cord. Absent in this situation was the most characteristic factor causing medullary trauma, namely intrusion of encroaching bone into the cord tissue at high speed. Rather, a momentary bending tensile stress had been set up in the cord of this patient; this effect disappeared as soon as the slipped atlas was reduced by cervical traction, which in this case could not cause any harm since there had obviously not been any intrinsic cord lesion. Somewhat the same is true in case 98, where 10 days after discontinuation of traction an unstable vertebrae redislocated and pressed on the cervical cord, thus setting up bending tensile stress within the cord. Such stress is characterized by relatively mild, short-range overstretching of axially oriented fibres in spinal pathways, which has proven to be quickly relieved when pressure of encroaching bone is eliminated [7]. Accordingly, in this patient the neurological consequences of this stress largely disappeared as soon as the vertebra in question had been restored to its normal position by stretching the posterior longitudinal ligament (no weight is mentioned in the clinical notes). Well-known parallels in neurological surgery include relievable symptoms produced by pressure on a cranial nerve (e.g. the optic nerve [42]) and a discal hernia on the spinal cord or a spinal nerve root (for examples see [7]).

As evidence to corroborate their claim that therapeutic skull traction can do no harm, neurologists and rehabilitation therapists have pointed to observations similar to those in the above cases 38 and 98, maintaining that traction had not altered the neurological condition of a patient or had even led to disappearance of his or her neurological symptoms. As the circumstances in cases 38 and 98 show, however, such observations only prove that the patients had suffered no substantial intrinsic cord lesion that could have been amplified by traction and thus could have given rise to persistent neurological symptoms.

In the first two patients in Table 10 skull traction was performed with the cervical spine dorsiflexed. (As shown in Fig. 1, the shortening of the cervical canal and cord thereby produced the expected results in slackening of the cervical cord.) According to their reports, the two therapists who had relaxed the injured cord by dorsiflexion of the cervical spine noted a remarkably early and comprehensive return of neurological functions in these patients. Compared with the results in the remaining 97% of patients, obtained by conventional skull traction with a straight cervical spine, the neurological improvement in these two patients was clearly superior and, as will be shown below, as such was also indicative of relaxation of the cervical cord.

The cord has also been visibly relaxed in the third patient in Table 10 (case 60), who had undergone open reduction of an ILF at the C-3/C-4 level, followed by cerclage of the C-2 to C-4/C-5 spinous processes (a measure that resulted in shortening of the cervical canal). The cord relaxation was expressly recorded by the surgeon, who at the end of the operation noted good pulsation of the cervical cord.

Table 10. Early return of neurological functions brought about by dorsiflexion of the cervical spine with resultant relaxation of the spinal cord

Case no.	Age (years)	Level of injury	Special measures	Traction (kg)	Entry in clinical records
18	24	C-5/C-6	"Neck moderately extended by pillow under shoulder blades."	6.9–3.2	"Dislocation reduced by next morning, traction reduced by 8 lb to 7 lbs. Probably ECRL (extensor carpi radialis longus) returned on both sides by the following day and plantar reflexes were intermittently flexor. By 20.6.72 (2 days later) sensation was returning in the UL and wrist movements had improved. There was subsequently improvement in both sensation and motor power in both upper limbs with return of biceps and triceps jerks." Dr. David Hancock, Stoke Mandeville Hospital
55	46	C-4/C-5	"Skeletal traction applied with the neck extended."	6.4	7 days after dorsiflexion of cervical spine: "The pain was beginning to increase in both arms and the legs were flaccid." 14 days after dorsiflexion: "At this time he had regained light touch and proprioception in his lower limbs and a sensory level (at C-5) was no longer detectable. He has also regained function of his wrist extensors and slight function of his wrist flexors." Dr. Stephen Karp, Westminster Hospital
6	25	C-3/C-4	"Wiring of C-2 to C-4/5 spinous processes."	20.7	(Since reduction of interlocked facets C-3/C-4 was not achieved by traction with 20.7 kg, open cerclage of C-2 to C-4/C-5 spinous processes was performed) "At the end of operation good pulsation of the cord was noted." "Postoperatively patient made recovery of sensations in arms and legs and posterior tract functions returned, though motor function did not improve." Hialeah Hospital, Florida

After a pair of Crutchfield tongs had fallen out at night, one patient, who had been on traction (1.8 kg) for 6 weeks, complained of discomfort in the right shoulder and of his inability to move his right arm and legs as before. An immediate check by the head of department showed no objective changes compared with neurological findings recorded 4 days previously; indeed, marked improvement of the functions in question had been recorded 2 days later. (The patient was a

38-year-old engineer with partial Brown-Séquard's paralysis resulting from an injury at the level of C-5/C-6; see case 25, Table 7).

As we know from experience, when skull traction is established after traumatic compression of the cervical cord, development of medullary oedema can contribute to increasing neurological deficit; the influence of possible oedema should therefore never be left out of consideration. On the other hand, there is no physiological factor so far known which could cause the marked neurological improvement recorded in certain cases shortly after termination of cervical traction other than cessation of the overstretching of surviving axis cylinders.

Addendum to Chapter 3: Recent Clinical Evidence

As this manuscript was ready to go to press, the author received reports of further observations corroborating its thesis, made on young patients with fresh cervical cord injury in whom traction had initially been established. Part of their neurological deficit regressed impressively quickly as soon as the calipers were removed and their cervical spine was released from traction.

The patients in whom these observations were made have been analysed at National Spinal Injuries Centre, Stoke Mandeville Hospital, Aylesbury, England, by Dr. Alison Graham[1], Senior House Officer, a colleague of Dr. John Silver, Consultant in Spinal Injuries. Dr. Silver commented upon these notes: "... Two patients never had traction at all and made a steady uneventful recovery but the other three, B ..., M ... and C ..., showed a dramatic improvement within 24 hours of removal of traction. I think these cases ... do illustrate that something dramatic happens upon removal of the traction to the neurophysiology of the spinal cord."

Case Histories

T.B., D.o.A.: 16 August 1987. 27-yr-old man, fell off a wall. Fracture of C-6 vertebra. Cone calipers traction inserted on day one. 8 lb traction applied. Neurology on day one: *R:* Trapezius, deltoid, biceps 4+, triceps 3, wrist flex and ext 3+. *L:* Trapezius, deltoid 4, triceps 3, biceps 4, wrist flex and ext 2. Legs *(R+L):* O; Plantar: downgoing. Reflex *(R+L):* B, T+, S−, Abdo−, K−, A−, Plantar *(R+L):* downgoing. Sensory: light touch preserved all segments, blunt below C-8 *(R+L)*, pin prick *R:* C-8, *L:* C-8. *Traction removed* on admission to Spinal Unit: within 24 h improvement; *R* arm: Trapezius 5, deltoid, biceps, triceps 4+, wrist flex and ext 4+, interossei 3+, *L* arm: Trapezius 5, biceps, triceps, deltoid, wrist 4+. *R* leg: no improvement in muscle power until 4 wks post injury, *L* leg: no improvement until 4 wks post injury. Sensory: 4 wks sensory level T-1, Reflex *(R+L):* B, T, S+, abdo−, K−, A−, plantar−. Plantar upgoing at 3 wks, hyperreflexic lower limbs at 3 wks.

P.M., D.o.A.: 17 January 1988. 19-yr-old man injured in RTA. Suffered fracture dislocation of C-5 on C-6. Gardner-Well traction inserted on day one of accident. 11 lb weight applied. Neurology on admission: *R:* Trapezius, deltoid, biceps, triceps 4, wrist flex and ext 3, intrinsic hand 2+. *L:* 4. Lower limb *(R+L):* 4. Reflex *(R+L):* B, T, S+, abdo+, K++, A++, plantar *(R+L):* upgoing. Sensory level: *R:* normal, *L:* hypaesthesia C-6/T-1. 18.01.88: *Transfer SMH.* Traction reduced each day 2 lb until 5 days post injury. *Traction removed:*

---

[1] Dr. Graham's valuable help is gratefully acknowledged.

Bladder function returned to normal within 24 h of removing traction. Marked improvement in power of *R* arm: all muscle groups within 24 h with return to normal power within 8 wks. *L* arm: improvement in 24 h of intrinsic hand muscles grade 3 to 4+; return to grade 5 within 2 wks. *R* leg: no change in neuro post removal; grade 5 power achieved within 6 wks. Reflex *(R+ L)* as before; plantar downgoing. Sensory level: dropping within 24 h of removal; normal sensation 6 wks post injury.

R.C., D.o.A.: 29 February 1988. 23-yr-old man, fell from roof, a distance of 20 feet. On admission to referring hospital he was found to have undisplaced compression fracture of C-3 and C-6. He also had a closed head injury so initial neurological examination was difficult. He did withdraw to pain. All tendon reflexes were present but diminished. *R* Plantar was equivocal and *L* was definitely downgoing. Gardner-Well tongs were inserted on day one of admission, 8 lb applied. 18.03.88: *Transfer SMH:* Neurologic picture by time of admission: *R:* Trapezius 5, deltoid 4+, supinator 4, triceps 4+, wrist flex and ext 4+, intrinsic hand 4+. *L:* Trapezius 5, deltoid 4, supinator 4, triceps 4, wrist flex and ext 1, intrinsic hand 1. All upper limb reflexes were present and normal. Abdominal reflexes were absent. Knee jerk on *R* and ankle jerk *R* absent. Knee and ankle jerk on *L* hyperreflexic. Both plantars were upgoing. Lower limb power on admission: *R* Adductor 2, *L* 0, *R* Ankle flex 2, *L* 0; *R* Ankle ext 0. Sensory level on admission: last normal segment *(R+ L):* C-6. *Traction removed on 24.03.88.* Bladder function returned 26.03.88. No dramatic change in neurology with removal of traction. Gradual slow recovery until 16.06.88, incomplete sensory level *(R+ L):* C-6. All lower limb reflexes hyperreflexic. Both plantars upgoing. Biceps and supinator reflexes both brisk bilaterally. Power returned: All muscle groups *R* arm normal (5), *L* arm all muscle groups 5 except intrinsic muscles hand (4+), *R* leg all muscle groups 4, *L* leg all muscle groups 3.

Comments and Discussion

As these notes show, traction was removed at different points of time: in the first patient after 24 h; in the second after 5 days, after stepwise reduction of the load - neurological functions did not return until all weight had been removed. Whilst reaction to removal was striking in these two patients, the third patient responded with no other conspicuous improvement than return of bladder function. In his case, however, traction was removed after 3 weeks and tetraparesis had been less marked than in the previous patients. This explains why the favourable reactions of this patient were less substantial and can hardly be characterized as dramatic (as also pointed out by the examiner).

These new observations at Stoke Mandeville Hospital have brought new evidence that motor power, control of bladder and other neurological functions can, after cancelling of skull traction, reappear relatively quickly and - as far as, e.g. bladder function is concerned - to a surprising degree of complexity. Neurological improvement of this kind is a real physiological event and not one expected in theory (i.e., an imagined one), as some earlier critics were at first prone to anticipate.

It was reassuring to see that bladder control in the SMH patients returned. This effect, equally important for patient and ward staff, has taken place in all patients treated so far by spinal cord relaxation. This is a decisive step forward in the care of paralysed patients that cannot be overestimated, since urinary incontinence is one of the most disabling symptoms that also is often life-endangering.

4 Cord Incision Model for Visualization of Adverse Effects of Skull Traction and Ventroflexion of Cervical Spine

A preliminary observation, illustrated in Fig. 9, is that skull traction straightens the cervical spine out of its normal lordosis, thus causing the surfaces of an incision (or wound) to move apart. The graphs in Fig. 10 show that this diastasis increases as the degree of skull traction or of ventroflexion of the neck is increased. Figure 11 presents measurements which make clear that lengthening of the spinal canal brought about by flexion of the cervical spine is additive to that produced by flexion of the (upper) thoracic spine [67, 68] and therefore increases the gaping of a transverse intramedullary wound. This additive effect of simultaneous skull traction and ventroflexion of the cervical spine is demonstrated in Fig. 12. From the biomechanical measurements available today it can be inferred that stretching of the straight cervical spinal cord by traction on the cervical spine reaches a maxi-

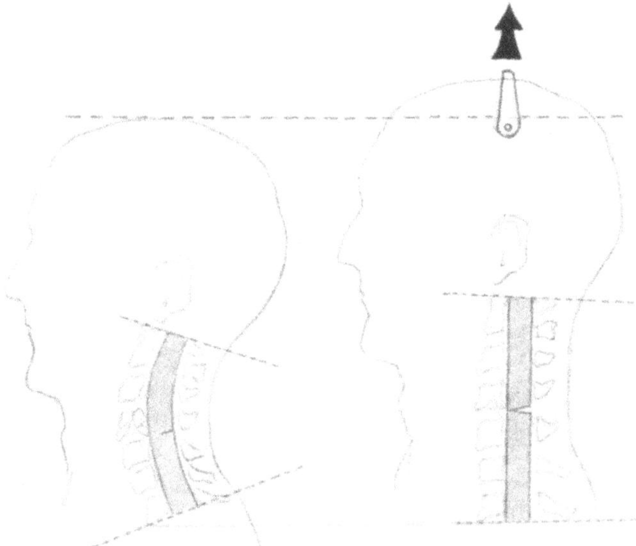

Fig. 9. Effects of skull traction on configuration of the neck. With the body prone and the skull immobilized (so that the chin cannot move either), skull traction with a force of only 4–5 kg straightens out the normal lordosis of the cervical spine so that the neck contour becomes plane and the head and neck are lifted up accordingly; the same straightening of the neck lordosis occurs with the body supine. At the moment when the cervical spine has become straight a very slight movement of the region of the incision can just be noticed (first indication of incipient retraction of the surfaces of this model wound on continuation of traction)

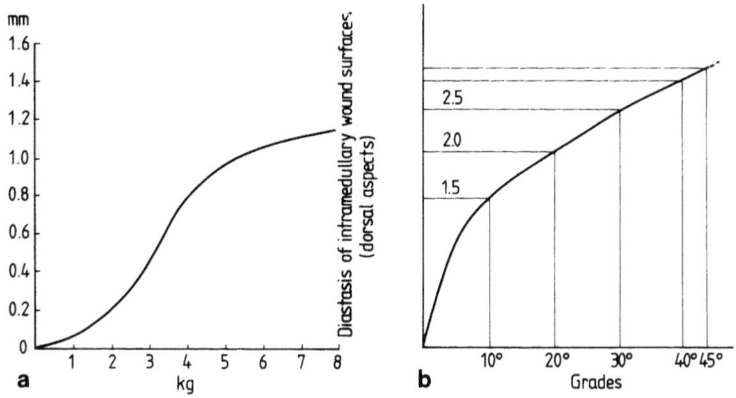

Fig. 10. **a** Approximate effects of skull traction on degree of diastasis of intramedullary wound surfaces viewed from the posterior aspect. **b** Approximate effects of flexion of cervical spine (from its erect posture to maximum ventroflexion) on diastasis of intramedullary wound surfaces viewed from the posterior aspect

mum when carried out with a load of about 7 kg, provided that no osseous, cartilaginous or ligamentous damage is present. As illustrated in Fig. 13, the width of the intramedullary wound cleft in the cervical cord increases with increasing length of the cervical canal (irrespective of its absolute length). As discussed above, this effect can be relatively greater in a patient with a short neck than in one with a long cervical spine. Figure 12 shows, moreover, that traction on the *straight* cervical spine has a relatively limited - and, in general, equal - distractive effect on the width of the intramedullary wound gap, whilst traction on the *ventroflexed* cervical spine leads to an increase in the width of the intramedullary wound gap, which widens with increasing ventroflexion, i.e. with lengthening of the cervical spinal column.

4.1 Thinned Section of Compressed Cervical Cord: Special Vulnerability to Abnormal Forces

As is known from surgical and pathological observations, the traumatically compressed area of the cervical cord after spinal injury has an irregular, approximately oval shape with borders sloping towards its centre [2, 7, 48]. To understand why and how the compressed cervical spinal cord can be further damaged by skull traction, a peculiar effect of traction on elastic bodies must be considered. If traction is exerted on an elastic body containing a thinned area in its substance, the material bordering on this thinned part is drawn out more than the rest of the body. This happens, for instance, if one stretches a rubber band, from the middle of which a quadrangular part has been cut out (Fig. 14): When the rubber band is stretched, the horizontal superior and inferior margins of the defect retract in a convex curve towards the superior and inferior sources of traction. An area of spinal cord that has been thinned and weakened by compression reacts similarly. The

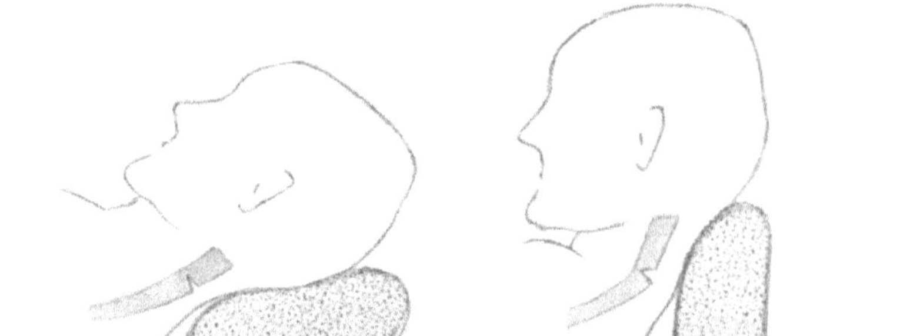

Fig. 11 a, b. Effects of neck posture and skull traction on compressive intramedullary wound visualized by transverse cord incision at C-6 level (manual traction with a force of 7 kg on a pair of Crutchfield tongs anchored in the acoustic meatus plane and controlled by a spring balance). **a** The surfaces of the transverse model wound at C-6 are drawn apart slightly when the cervical spine is moderately ventroflexed *(left)*, and more markedly when it is flexed to a higher degree *(right)*. (Note the significance of the different head supports.) **b** The amounts of gaping of the wound surfaces of the incision at C-6 (indicated by Arabic numerals along the arcs) brought about by traction with a constant load of 7 kg and spinal flexion of 10°, 20°, 30° and 45° at the upper thoracic level (approximately at the apex of the triangle). The amounts of gaping of the wound surfaces of the transverse incision produced by the same constant load but with increased ventroflexion of the spine (at the upper thoracic level) are seen at the intersections of the radiuses with the inner arc. The amounts of gaping of the C-6 incision produced by the same tractive load and the same thoracic flexion but with additional ventroflexion of the cervical spine at the mid-cervical level (as shown in **a**, *right*) are shown at intersections of the radiuses with the outer arc

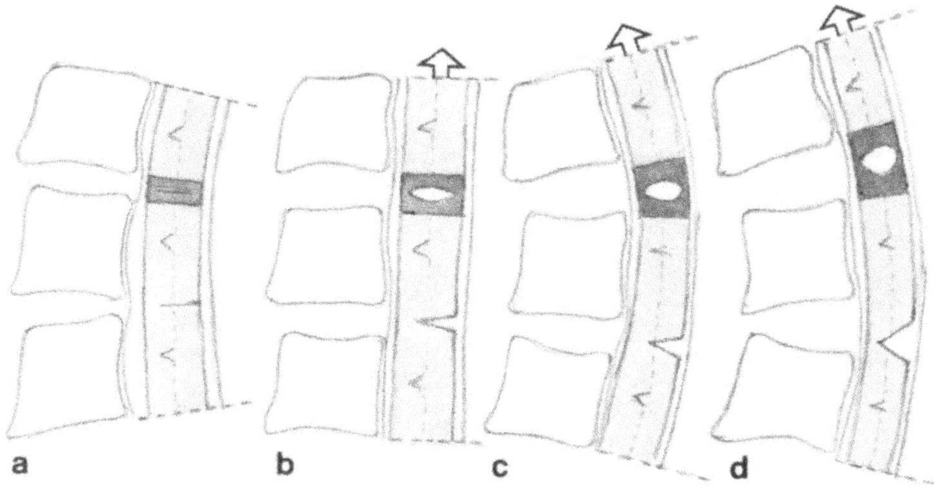

Fig. 12a–d. The lower two-thirds of the cord model demonstrates the effects of therapeutic skull traction on a transverse intramedullary wound comprising the posterior two-thirds of the cervical cord (increase in height of intervertebral discs exaggerated). **a** Section of cervical spine and cord unloaded. Wound surfaces in close contact with each other (favoured by physiological lordosis of cervical spine). **b** Therapeutic traction with the cervical spine straight has stretched the cervical cord elastically; the intramedullary wound surfaces are slightly drawn apart. **c** Traction with the same force as in **b** but with the cervical spine moderately ventroflexed: stretching by traction has been added to its physiological stretching on ventroflexion; the intramedullary wound opens in a wedge shape (as also in **b**), since the surfaces are further apart dorsally than ventrally. **d** On traction with the cervical spine maximally flexed, the gaping of the intramedullary wound has increased maximally, since the amount of elastic stretching of the cord due to traction and that due to ventroflexion of the cervical spine are additive. The upper third of the cord model shows the retraction/deformation of the surfaces of a transverse compressive intramedullary wound within the centre of the cord (*dark zone*, **a–d**), brought about by therapeutic skull traction with the same load

effect is essentially the same when, in order to represent a thinned and weakened but still continuous part of the compressed cervical cord, the rectangular defect is reinforced by a piece of rubber sheet that is only slightly thinner than the rest of the rubber band.

This model demonstrates clearly that it is just the area containing thinned and weakened nerve fibres that, on cervical traction, is subjected to more intensive stretching than the medullary tissue of ordinary thickness surrounding it. This mechanism can only lead to further impairment and possibly to ultimate rupturing of weakened, axially oriented nerve fibres and blood vessels.

4.2 Cumulative Adverse Effects of Traction and Ventroflexion

Tension generated in the medullary tissue by therapeutic traction is bound to increase the extent of damage to the medullary tissue, not only within the thinned, weakened section of the cervical cord, as just described, but also in tissue border-

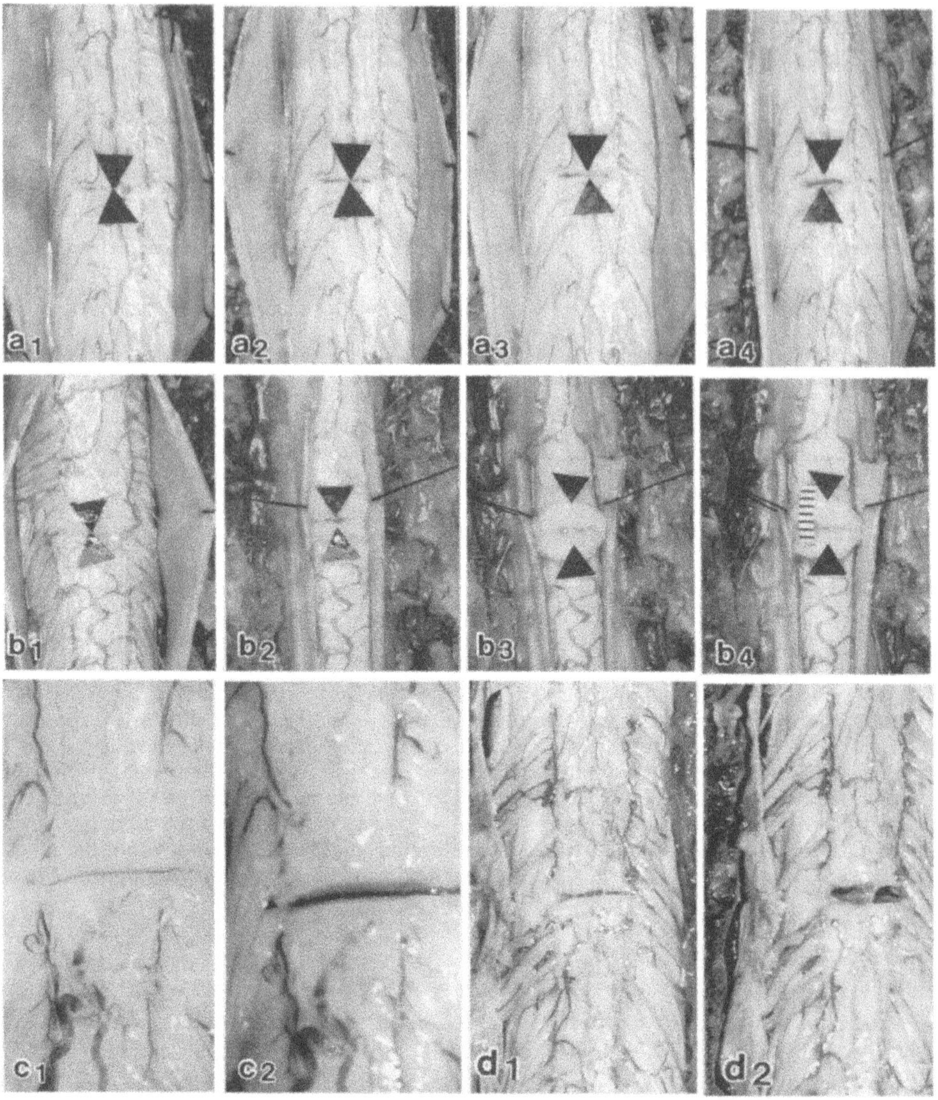

Fig. 13a–d. Effects of skull traction on transverse incisions at C-5/C-6 levels in the cervical cord, representing traumatic cord ruptures, in four cadavers in the prone position. Traction on the cervical spine exerted by a pair of Crutchfield tongs, anchored in the parietal bone and loaded by approximately 6 kg in all specimens (spring balance control).
$\mathbf{a}_1, \mathbf{b}_1, \mathbf{c}_1, \mathbf{d}_1$ Spine unloaded (note: depth of transverse incision smallest in **a**, greatest in **c**). $\mathbf{a}_2, \mathbf{b}_2, \mathbf{c}_2, \mathbf{d}_2$ Spine under traction. In $\mathbf{a}_2$ and $\mathbf{b}_2$ (with shallow incisions) the *black indicators* have moved apart slightly; in $\mathbf{c}_2$ and $\mathbf{d}_2$ (with deep incisions) the wound surfaces have moved apart markedly. In $\mathbf{b}_2$ the dura mater, by stretching, has moved mediad, thus obscuring lateral aspects of the cord. $\mathbf{a}_3, \mathbf{b}_3$ Spine under traction and ventroflexed through 5°. In $\mathbf{a}_3$ separation of the *indicators* is more marked than without spinal flexion; in $\mathbf{b}_3$ pulp has protruded over pial surfaces. $\mathbf{a}_4, \mathbf{b}_4$ Spine under traction and ventroflexion through 10°. In $\mathbf{a}_4$ and $\mathbf{b}_4$ the *indicators* have moved further apart and the stretched dura has moved mediad; in $\mathbf{b}_4$ (as also in $\mathbf{b}_3$) an incision had to be made into the dura blades bilaterally to render traction effects on cord visible

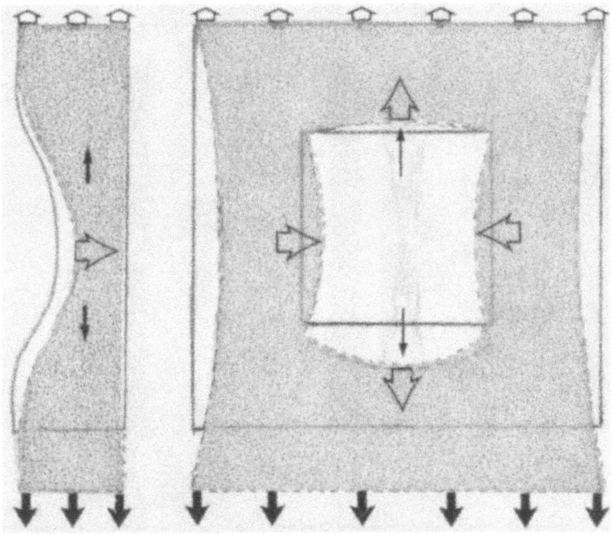

Fig. 14. Effect of vertical stretching on a rubber band from which a rectangular area has been cut out and replaced by a slighly thinner rubber sheet. The weakened part is subjected to more intensive stretching than the surrounding material of normal thickness

ing on a *partial* transverse cord rupture (and the majority of ruptures are partial): the surfaces of such an intramedullary wound are drawn apart so much that weakened nerve fibres around the corner of the wound come under the influence of notch stresses. (In the presence of a cleft in any material, traction on the material generates notch stress in the neighbourhood of this cleft; cf. [7, 18] and Fig. 15. In practice, notch stress implies increased tension in nerve fibres and blood vessels bordering on the edge of an intramedullary gap.) With a growing number of distended or ruptured nerve fibres during traction treatment of injured patients, the degree of conductivity of the cervical cord is thus reduced and the neurological deficit proportionally increased. The distortion effect is likely to occur after cervical traction has been started, whereas rupturing has probably most often already happened at the moment of compressive impact on the cord.

Repetition of an experiment is generally laborious and unrewarding. However, if the adverse biomechanical influence of spinal traction should be doubted, it is an easy task - and more than worthwhile in view of the implications for correct treatment of patients with spinal injuries - to look at a transverse incision in the cervical cord of a fresh human cadaver and to check the influences of dorsi- and ventroflexion of the neck on the surfaces of this wound. Even if no traction has been applied to the cervical spine, these surfaces invariably retract from each other and open to a fairly large gap when the head is only slightly ventroflexed.

Today, this effect is evident from an ever increasing number of clinical observations. From these, it appears extremely likely that this adverse mechanism affects an unfortunately large number of patients with spinal lesions. As shown by the dramatic events described below, it suffices even to place a cushion under the injured patient's head: this stretches the cervical cord enough to induce retraction of

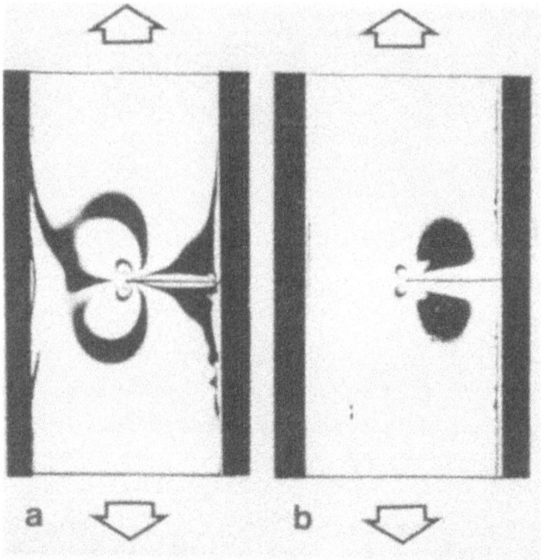

Fig. 15 a, b. Notch stress visualized photoelastically in Araldite plates with horizontal incisions on the *right*. **b** Araldite plate reinforced by two Araldite plates glued to its front and back. **a, b** Plates exposed to traction *(arrows)*. Reactive forces in the material bordering on the clefts are recorded photoelastically. Isochromes in plate **a**, indicating reactive forces in its material, are spread over a larger area than those in the sandwiched plate **(b)**; however, despite its double reinforcement, traction produced reactive forces in this plate also. It is concluded from these observations that even undamaged nerve fibres bordering on a transverse intramedullary rupture are exposed to tensile stress, even when covered by undamaged pia mater spinalis

the surfaces of any transverse intramedullary wound and stretches thinned and weakened nerve fibres in the traumatically compressed cervical cord.

In one of our patients with a cervical medullary lesion (a woman aged 58 years, treated at the Red Cross Hospital, Stockholm) we performed surgical fixation of the cervical spine in slight dorsiflexion by means of a tibial bone graft implanted ventrally into vertebral bodies C-3 to C-7. Three days after surgery, when the sensibility in the perianal region was already recovering, and the vesical and anal sphincteric functions were improving, a cushion put under the patient's head during the night by an uninformed nurse - moving the neck into no more than just the erect posture - instantly reversed these improvements. The cause of this sudden neurological deterioration was, of course, that the slight forward bending of the patient's head and cervical spine caused the transplant to lift from its track - a fact confirmed later radiographically - and the cervical cord to be very slightly stretched. This observation strikingly documents the sensitivity of damaged nerve fibres in cervical cord pathways to even minor stretching. In this patient the adverse effects of cord stretching became especially evident as the recovering neurological functions were suddenly suppressed. In patients with a fresh compressive cord injury, stretching of the cord by skull traction is obviously even more marked. But since in their cases the neurological functions are declining, the deleterious effects of traction are not as clearly evident.

In the light of such saddening experiences there can scarcely be any doubt that the recently widespread recommendation that "if traction is used, the neck should be slightly flexed" [24, 23] is bound to inflict additional serious damage to the cervical cord of patients who are treated in this way, leaving them with life-long disability. It is to be hoped that the facts presented here will motivate our readers to join the present efforts to ban skull traction from modern rehabilitation.

4.3 Hyperextension Injury to Cervical Cord: Biomechanical Factors

In our experimental studies on the effects of spinal cord compression we did not reproduce all conditions prevailing in hyperextension injuries to the cervical cord. In a conceivable model the cervical canal should be narrowed by having a dowel pushed into it anteriorly through a burrhole in vertebrae C-5/C-6 (where, according to statistics, cord damage most frequently occurs [58, 59]) to represent an osteophyte. From observations of the effects of cord compression in ventroflexed, erect and dorsiflexed postures of the cervical spine, however, we have obtained the following conception of the biomechanical factors in a hyperextension injury. On extension of the cervical spine the cervical cord is relaxed and its tissue thrown into folds (see Fig. 1); this phenomenon results in an increase in the cross-section (overall thickening) of the cervical spinal cord. Added to this, during extension of the cervical spine the lumen of the cervical canal is further reduced by folding of the dura and ligamenta flava bulging into the cervical canal. It is therefore probable that, in an accident in which the cervical spine is abruptly hyperextended, the sudden constriction in the lumen of the canal renders the osteophyte at the anterior wall of the narrowed cervical canal just as harmful as a loose bone fragment intruding into the spinal cord at high speed [47]. The osteophyte against which medullary tissue is suddenly pressed thus has the effect of a moving pincer head, squeezing forth viscous pulp craniad and caudad with resultant thinning, weakening and, possibly, rupturing of the cervical cord [61].

Circumstances which can account for the observation that traumatic compression of the dorsiflexed cord is neurologically often less disabling than compression of the cord in ventroflexed postures of the cervical spine are probably related to the fact that, in an extended/shortened cord, axis cylinders and blood vessels are relaxed. As verified in the above experiments, there is thus a certain margin before they are stretched to an extent just as deleterious in effect as a bone fragment rapidly encroaching upon the cervical cord with the spine in an erect or ventroflexed posture. Another fact is that cord compression in a hyperextension injury often takes place at a lower speed than in the majority of compressive accidents with a straight or ventroflexed cervical spine.

Also, after a hyperextension injury of the cervical cord the cervical spine must be kept in slight dorsiflexion to relax damaged cord tissue and to avoid injurious effects of even slight ventroflexion. For reasons discussed above, the injudicious recommendation that patients with a hyperextension injury should be treated by traction and ventroflexion of the cervical spine [24] must be strongly condemned, since these measures are bound to lead to serious neurological deficit in such patients [7].

4.3.1 Extrusion of Soft Pulp Contributing to Medullary Damage

Of the multitude of structures involved in the important and fascinating effect of automatic lengthening and shortening of the spinal cord, the rhombic meshwork of connective tissue fibres in the outer layer of the pia mater spinalis participates in and promotes a special pathological phenomenon.

As has been shown since 1960 [6], upon elastic elongation of the cord, starting from the erect posture, the cranial and caudal angles of intersection of the connective tissue fibres become progressively narrower to a certain predetermined angle, whereas on shortening of the cord they become wider. Accordingly, during elastic stretching of the cord on cervical traction or ventroflexion, the whole pia cylinder is narrowed (as is apparent from the reduced cross-sectional area of the cord; see Fig. 2), whereby its connective tissue mesh exerts pressure on the medullary pulp. As is visible at the borders of a model wound in the cervical cord (for example, as produced by a transverse incision into the cord), through this constriction a certain amount - usually very small - of viscous medullary pulp is squeezed forth, so that the inferior and superior surfaces of the transverse intramedullary wound bulge slightly. From this phenomenon it may be inferred that, after transverse rupturing of the cervical cord due to a compressive injury, cervical traction will inevitably have a similar, or possibly even greater, effect since in compressive injury the pia cylinder usually remains intact [7]. Possible additional damage exerted on the medullary tissue by constriction of the pia cylinder has not yet been studied. From our ealier observations on the effects of artificial spinal cord oedema it may be anticipated, however, that this phenomenon aggravates adverse intramedullary effects of post-traumatic oedema [7].

The fact that the surfaces of a transverse model wound bulge slightly, but increasingly, on increased stretching of the cord, is one reason why measurements of the width of the gap of the model wound cannot be exact. This holds true especially when, after repeated flexion-extension movements combined with traction on the cervical spine, a certain small amount of protruded pulp may have collected on the originally more or less smooth surfaces of the model wound. The width of the gap of this wound can then no longer be taken as an exact measurement; instead, when reliable data are required, it is advisable to make a new incision in the cord of a fresh cadaver.

5 Future Treatment of Cervical Spine Injuries

5.1 High Incidence of Disability Probably Caused by Concealed Effects of Cervical Traction

The deleterious effects of a prolonged mechanical load, as in the case of long-term cervical traction, on weakened medullary tissue have long remained hidden and difficult to uncover. With better acquaintance with the injurious potential of skull traction today one must be aware that this can aggravate and perpetuate the primary mechanical damage to the spinal cord tissue. It would therefore not be surprising if it turned out that, during the years of its unquestioned application, this treatment had caused additional, avoidable disability in numerous victims of spinal cord injury. Now that these effects have been demonstrated, appropriate measures must be taken to remove this procedure from clinical treatment [23] and to replace it with one aimed at stabilizing a damaged cervical spine by innocuous surgical and/or conservative orthopaedic methods.

5.2 Place of Traction in Future Reconstructive Spinal Surgery

During future cervical surgery and orthopaedic measures to stabilize an injured cervical spine, the head and spine will still have to be balanced and immobilized. This is not possible, of course, without temporary application of forces with tractive components to the head and cervical spine. As demonstrated in this study, when applied to the spine of a patient with a fresh spinal cord injury, traction should be limited, however, to a low grade (about 0.5-1 kg), and it would seem wise to keep the period of traction as short as possible. Admittedly, it is known today that undamaged nerve fibres which have been under pathological tension for months or even years can start conducting again when released from the load in question [7, 28, 35, 39, 46, 66], but for substantially damaged and weakened nerve fibres, the conductivity of which can be irreversibly destroyed by even short-term stretching, the duration and degree of stretching are highly significant.

Today, stabilization of the cervical spine can be achieved by bone transplants and extrinsic as well as intracorporeal splints and screws. In 1978 we devised a steel-frame prosthesis for bridging one or two crushed cervical vertebrae from the front, by cementing its upper and lower horizontal processes into the vertebral bodies of undamaged vertebrae above and below the fractured one [7]. Three or four vertebrae joined in this fashion are then immobilized in light dorsiflexion. This technique, supplemented by CLD, allowed two patients with a fractured cervical vertebra to be sat up as early as a few days after the operation [7].

However, the most recent development in modern orthopaedics is the stabilization of fractured cervical vertebrae by rigid internal screw fixation [5, 44, 49, 50, 52]. This technique makes it possible to dispense with skull traction and the likewise dangerous halopelvic immobilization. As with the above-mentioned prosthetic method, the patient can be seated within a few days of the injury. An important innovation which may possibly make screw fixation techniques even more attractive in the future is the introduction of titanium as material for screws (the screws being provided with hollow spaces to allow ingrowth of osteoblasts), as used by Morscher for physiological osteo-integration [49]. It seems likely that this will minimize the previously relatively high rate of infection and secondary instability after spinal screw fixation.

Irrespective of whether the (today mandatory) mechanical stabilization of the cervical spine is secured by bone splints, metacrylic bridges, titanium screws or splints of biodegradable polymeric compounds, prior to or during application of these means tools such as Crutchfield tongs will in the future still have to be applied for a short period. However, their use must be modified. The neck, for example, can be held slightly reclined over a round bolster, with the Crutchfield tongs anchored in the anterolateral aspect of the frontal bone and loaded with only 0.5-1 kg to keep the cervical spine and head in this position. During turning manoeuvres it is sufficient to secure this posture by a plastic semicollar, for instance, to support the chin and anterior aspect of the neck.

5.3 Outlook for New Methods to Promote Biological Healing

In patients with a cervical spinal cord injury, therapeutic efforts should, of course, be directed primarily towards restoration and maintenance of cord conductivity. Today, efforts to increase our still imperfect understanding of the nature of the damage caused to nerve fibres in spinal pathways and of optimal biomechanical conditions for their healing are largely replaced by measures for establishing an acceptable outer appearance of the cervical spine. Many a traumatic spinal deformity could certainly be accepted if only the capacity of the cervical cord for transmission had been saved, and if the spinal deformity in question were stable, so that during the normal range of movements it could not exert injurious pressure on the cervical cord [33].

As this study demonstrates, it is an error to assume that therapeutic traction protects the cervical cord from further damage. Contrary to the beliefs supporting the obsolete traction concept, it is clear that minor movements in the frontal plane of both the spine and the cervical cord - which have hitherto been feared - can be regarded as absolutely innocuous as long as the cervical cord is relaxed. As shown above, relaxation of the spinal cord commences at the moment when the cervical spine is only slightly dorsiflexed. In its relaxed state, even the traumatized cervical cord is surprisingly insusceptible to movements in the horizontal plane. We have demonstrated this fact in, among others, a patient with a C-2/C-3 intramedullary tumour, which could easily be extirpated by drawing the relaxed encasing medullary tissue aside after the cervical spine had been slightly dorsiflexed [7]. The innocuousness of this procedure was strikingly confirmed by the fact that, immediately after extubation the patient resumed spontaneous breathing, and that shortly afterwards sensibility and power in the arms and legs improved, the pain regressed and (a week later) bladder control recovered.

The clinical experience at Aylesbury has impressively confirmed the potential of therapeutic relaxation of the spinal cord: major early neurological improvements were recorded exclusively in patients whose cervical cord had been relaxed by dorsiflexion of the cervical spine. This strongly indicates that future active surgical treatment of patients with spinal cord injuries should be based on the principles of the new surgical measure - CLD - which we have developed in recent years [13, 18, 20, 21]. After this simple and economical intervention the cervical spine is permanently held in slight dorsiflexion by transcutaneous fixation of the lower part of the parietal bone to the upper thoracic spinous processes (see Figs. 18, 21). Both in patients with acute and in those with chronic spinal cord injury this procedure has resulted in convincing neurological improvements; this has also been the case at Aylesbury, where (on our recommendation) the dorsiflexion effect has been tested by a surgeon.

5.4 Inadvisability of Skull Traction in Treatment of Patients with Cervical Cord Injury

5.4.1 Factors Bearing on Deleterious Effects of Cervical Traction

The degree of harmfulness of the effects of cervical traction on an injured spinal cord is dependent on the following factors:

1. The extent of medullary destruction (deleterious effects of traction, inevitable).
   - The presence of numerous compressed and weakened nerve fibres in functionally important spinal pathways with exhausted resistance to normal elastic stretching, which are accordingly disposed to increased thinning and rupturing under tractive load.
   - An increasing degree of ventroflexion of the cervical and/or upper thoracic spine, irrespective of the level of the ventroflexion.
2. Constitutional factors (deleterious effects, highly probable).
   - A relatively short cervical canal in persons with a slim skeletal build.
   - The combination of a short neck (short vertebral bodies) with a relatively high degree of integrated yielding of neck tissue (intervertebral discs, ligaments and muscles). (Since the strength of the cervical cord is proportional to the length of the bony vertebral canal, increased yielding of soft tissues exposes a relatively short cervical cord to a relatively marked degree, i.e. distance, of stretching.)
3. Acquired defects of cervical structures (deleterious effects, relatively probable).
   - Fractures of vertebral bones, making the upper and lower parts of damaged vertebrae liable to be pulled apart in axial directions.
4. Traumatic ruptures of discs and ligaments, allowing pathological distraction of vertebrae, as above (deleterious effects, relatively probable).

- Weakness of cervical column due to osteoporosis, sequelae of rheumatoid arthritis, weak cervicothoracic structures, a weak muscle girdle, etc. (deleterious effects relatively improbable).

5.4.2 Discussion and Demonstration

Publications describing the transverse intramedullary wound as a regular consequence of any marked compression of the spinal cord [7, 21, 61] have obviously not yet reached all professionals engaged in treatment of patients with spinal injuries.

To hasten abandonment of skull traction and its replacement by other stabilizing orthopaedic procedures we sought to demonstrate its adverse effects on an artificial compressive wound in the cervical cord of a living animal. At length, we got an opportunity to show these effects in an anaesthetized cat (Department of Physiology, University of Gothenburg, 1985). After laminectomy at an upper thoracic level, the plunger of a plastic syringe was held resting on the dura and given a swift blow with a tablespoon. The plunger was immediately lifted, and a marked transverse crack in the cord was visible through the translucent dura (Fig. 16). For extraneous reasons, traction could not be applied in this cat. However, the mechanical effect of skull traction on a ruptured or transected cord is apparent from

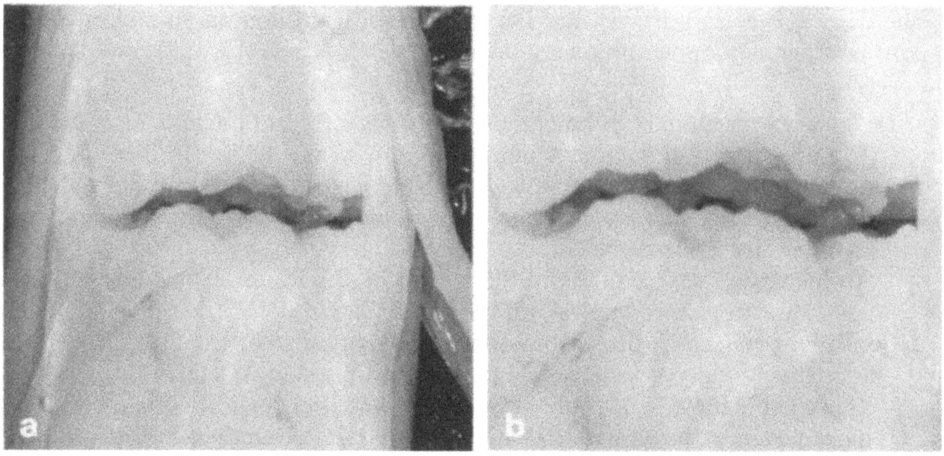

Fig. 16 a, b. Vital feline spinal cord reacting to in situ compression in the same way as a patient's cord injured in an accident, i.e. by rupturing transversely (cf. Figs. 4, 7, 8). In an anaesthetized cat, after laminectomy the plunger of a disposable syringe was held resting vertically on the translucent upper thoracic dura and a swift blow was delivered on its upper end with a tablespoon. Immediately a marked transverse fissure was visible through the dura. The cleft illustrated was preserved by formaldehyde perfusion through the cardiac route. (In the dog and cat spinal cord, with the animal in a prone, straight posture, there is obviously enough residual tension to produce marked gaping of the cleft [18].) (Specimen prepared at Institutes of Physiology and Neurobiology, University of Gothenburg; photo: Lars Mila, Carl Zeiss Svenska AB)

other observations: some experimenters performing studies on rats checked the occurrence of total transection of the spinal cord simply by exerting a pull simultaneously at the head and tail of the animal, so that if the cord had been totally transected, the stumps would be seen to move apart [32].

Hence, any orthopaedist or worker in the field of rehabilitation of patients with spinal injuries can today easily form a personal idea of the effect of skull traction - either in the human cadaver or in the experimental rat - and become familiar with its adverse effects on the injured spinal cord. (See a description of the transverse intramedullary fissure in the cervical cord produced by compression of the cord in 22 fresh human cadavers [7].)

6 Summary of Part I

6.1 Review and Discussion

In a score of operations a number of years ago using of a self-adjusting headrest designed for inducing various degrees of either stretching or relaxation of the spinal cord [7], we confirmed, firstly, that even very slight and often scarcely observable dorsiflexion of the cervical spine is sufficient to relax the entire spinal cord, and, secondly, that pulsation of the relaxed cervical cord stops immediately as soon as the cervical spine has assumed the erect posture, and elastic stretching of the (cervical) cord thus takes place. As has been shown here, it is the stretching of the injured cervical cord - more precisely of the thinned, weakened nerve fibres in the compressed section - that upsets the conductivity. There is thus much evidence that stretching of the injured section of the cervical cord inevitably results in neurological deficit. When therapeutic traction is applied to a damaged cervical cord, the conductivity of which has been suddenly reduced by the compressive injury, it obviously may be difficult to discern the consequently increasing neurological deficit from the range of various decreasing neurological functions. Seen from this perspective, the assumption that the percentage of recorded cases of neurological deficit among the SMH patients is far too low seems to be well based.

Our observations on experimental cord lesions made evident that contrary to a widespread clinical view, thinning and/or rupturing of the compressed cervical cord seldom comprises its entire cross-sectional area. Moreover, in spinal cross-sections compressed (weakened) areas are likely to appear as patches with irregular, fringed contours and to occupy various sites of the cross-sectional area. There is also neurological evidence that, within a compressed region of the cervical cord, a relatively large number of either complete pathways or bundles of such pathways must have remained basically intact and thus contain conductive nerve fibres. It is these weakened but surviving fibres that can be further damaged when exposed to overstretching during skull traction.

In the case of certain patients with clear-cut neurological symptoms and radiologically visible abnormalities, it is already possible today to determine the area within the cord cross-section where reactive intramedullary forces have caused overstretching of bundles of axons - from the direction, depth and speed of intrusion of the constricting body (usually bone) and other factors. This proved true in two of our former patients, in whom the approximate size, site and depth of intrusion of a bone fragment into the cervical canal/cord could be reconstructed from radiographs; the neurological symptoms in these patients corresponded fairly well with those predicted on the basis of these data [7].

We originally demonstrated the adverse effects of cervical traction in only a relatively small number of patients but were then able to corroborate them in the

Aylesbury records of 100 patients treated by skull traction. Our findings thus serve as a challenge to all workers in the field of rehabilitation. With the present, relatively ample documentation of this matter, the previous hesitation of these experts should now give way as they begin to replace skull traction with innocuous methods for adequate stabilization of the injured cervical spine.

To elucidate the potential deleterious effects of skull traction on an injured cervical cord, various methods have been utilized in the present study to illustrate the fact that reactive forces in the cervical cord are concentrated predominantly on its thinned section, where axially oriented nerve fibres and capillaries are distended and thus can be additionally damaged. In an attempt to shed light on the mechanism underlying this conception, basic effects of the compression of inanimate physical bodies were investigated. The biomechanics of the spinal cord was then considered, since many workers in the field of rehabilitation seem to be insufficiently familiar with this aspect or to pay inadequate consideration to it.

Three main methods were used to demonstrate the potential harmful effects of cervical traction. The first, indirect, method (Sect. 2) was to perform objective measurements on the length of the cervical canal in various physiological postures of the cervical spine. It was found that the cervical canal is elongated to a medium extent in the erect posture of the cervical spine. To the different degrees of elongation observed in various individuals an empirically derived value of 10 mm was added as a measure of the average elongation of the cervical canal during skull traction. From the figures obtained it was concluded that the cervical cord must stretch elastically to adapt itself to this increase in the length of the canal. For physical reasons discussed above, the detrimental effect of this stretching of the cervical cord is focused primarily on injured, thinned and weakened medullary tissue.

The second method (Sect. 3) consisted of collecting information about possible adverse effects of skull traction on an injured cervical cord. Clinical reports were scrutinized at centres providing specialist care on tetraplegic patients who at an early stage of their injury had been treated by skull traction. These patient records were examined over the period of time which was considered adequate in relation to the nature and degree of the spinal trauma. The results of this analysis show indisputably the extent to which therapeutic skull traction either increases the width of the defect in the cervical cord tissue caused by cord compression or increases the distension of its traumatically weakened section. They therefore provide a solid basis for an understanding of the way in which skull traction can potentially cause further damage to injured cervical spinal cord.

As a third method (Sect. 4), the characteristic transverse intramedullary wound (brought about in living vertebrates by compression of the cervical cord; see Fig. 16) was reproduced by transverse incision into the cervical cord in a score of fresh human cadavers. By applying traction with increasing loads it was clearly demonstrated in this model that the width of the transverse intramedullary rupture increases with increasing load on the skull traction device and hence on the cervical cord. Similarly, any traumatically thinned and weakened cord section reacts to increasing skull traction forces with increased thinning and possible ultimate rupturing (though not by an identical mechanism, see above). For these reasons it is logical to suppose that skull traction with a greater weight produces increasing medullary damage, reflected by aggravated neurological deficit.

The results of our analyses can be summarized succinctly in terms of the following points:

- Therapeutic traction is dangerous to an injured cervical spinal cord.
- Swift traumatic cord compression squeezes decomposed mucous medullary tissue caudad and craniad within the pia cylinder from the site of constriction.
- Compressed cervical cord is thinned; at a certain rate of constriction a transverse rupture (cleft) arises in the zone of maximum thinning.
- Upon skull traction traumatically weakened axis cylinders and blood vessels in the constricted cord section are stretched more than the surrounding medullary tissue (due to the general behaviour of elastic bodies).
- Traction draws apart wound surfaces of traumatic medullary clefts, thus aggravating the injury. Analogously, a surgeon would not draw apart a cut instead of suturing it.
- Traction promotes growth of glial and connective tissue into traumatic medullary clefts by widening the clefts.
- Ventroflexion of the head worsens the deleterious effects of cervical traction on thinned cervical cord by increasing the degree of stretching of still continuous tissue and those on transversely ruptured medullary tissue by drawing apart the surfaces of the respective transverse intramedullary wound clefts.
- Skull traction is more dangerous to the cervical cord of short-necked persons than to that of those with a long neck. By analogy, if a short and a long rubber band are stretched by the same amount, the edges of a nick in the short band will be drawn farther apart and more vigorously than those of a nick in the long rubber band.
- On application of therapeutic cervical traction in persons with fresh cervical spinal cord lesions, certain remaining conductive capabilities of the cervical cord disappear some time after the establishment of skull traction (recorded in about 12% of injured persons in the present investigation).

6.2 Conclusions

The intramedullary effects of compressive cervical injury are now clear and can be described as short-range deleterious overstretching of medullary tissue.

When substantial traction is applied to an injured cervical spine and spinal cord, in order to reduce the dislocation of a bone fragment that is pressing on the cervical cord and hence stretching it locally, the degree of overstretching of the compressed and thinned section of the cervical cord is increased. It is clear from this effect that skull traction is a potentially destructive force.

With knowledge of this now proven danger of therapeutic traction, medical workers both at the scene of accidents and in hospital care are again confronted with an old problem, namely the need to keep dislocated vertebral fragments or a whole vertebra immobile - prior to their surgical fixation - so that they or it cannot further encroach upon a damaged cervical cord. For this purpose a slight pull on the head or cervical spine with a maximum force of 1 kg is necessary to secure temporary immobilization both of the cervical spine and the impinging fragment.

As is well known, immobility of a fractured cervical spine can, moreover, be maintained by sand bags, by L-shaped soft plastic splints for fixation of the lateral aspect of the head and cervical spine and by semicollars for the anterior part of the neck, etc. When dislocated fractured bone has been either removed or immobilized in a position where it can no longer exert local pressure on the cord, it is advisable to maintain the lordosis of the cervical spine by a soft support fitting into its concavity; this ensures that straightening of the spine is prevented - a position in which cervical traction begins to have a deleterious effect on an injured cervical cord. This effect is potentiated by the addition of even slight ventroflexion to therapeutic traction.

In the case of ILF, skull traction with a force of about 7 kg can be sufficient to reduce the dislocation without doing any harm, provided that it is carried out during marked dorsiflexion of the cervicothoracic spine. This latter posture will bring about slackening of the spinal cord and thus protect its compressed - and hence overstretched - section from further damage. To allow sufficient dorsiflexion of the cervical spine during this combined postural reduction-traction manoeuvre, a broad support should be placed under the patient's upper thoracic spine. As is evident from Table 8, this measure can succeed in reducing ILF without causing increased damage to the injured cervical spinal cord.

With the present perspectives on cervical spinal cord injury, which emphasize the need for removal of conventional cervical traction from the therapeutic field, surgical methods for extirpation of fragments from the cervical canal by the anterior or anterolateral approach are again becoming of major importance. For patients in whom extirpation of such fragments is not considered, a multitude of histocompatible splints or screws are available today for reliable stabilization of the cervical spine (cf. p. 48). As confirmed by the well-known article published by the senior medical staff of SMH in 1969 [33], failure to reduce dislocations and fractures, or as we prefer to see it, acceptance of such conditions when harmless, does not rule out the possibility of excellent neurological recovery.

During the surgery mentioned above, use of traction with about 1 kg is unavoidable to keep the patient's head balanced and his cervical spine straight. Once the cervical cord is freed, for example, from pressure of dislocated bone, further injurious effects on the compressive intramedullary cord wound should be prevented by keeping the patient's cervical spine in slight lordosis.

Even if traction is used in the future, for a short period and on a much reduced scale, its force must be adjusted to the relative length of the patient's cervical spine and to the size of its vertebral bodies so that the risk of overstretching the traumatized cord section can be avoided.

As shown by the strikingly favourable neurological results in three SMH patients (Table 8) following relaxation of the cervical spinal cord and by the similarly beneficial outcome in a number of own patients upon whom we had operated with the CLD relaxation technique [7], the possibilities of restoring cord conductivity can today be basically improved by making use of this simple biological effect. For this reason, it would be a misconception to believe that the standard of rehabilitation already attained is so high that it cannot be surpassed. The fact, as documented in this work, that a significantly higher degree of neurological improvement has been achieved in patients whose cervical cord has been relaxed by surgically secured slight dorsiflexion of the cervical spine points to the likelihood that neurological functions can be restored to a much greater extent than is generally anticipated.

We now have the exciting prospect that, once the outdated traction therapy has been abandoned and replaced by surgical measures to slacken a damaged cervical cord, an improved prognosis for patients with spinal injuries is within reach. This would mean that the number of patients who are confined to a wheelchair would decrease substantially, and that, ultimately, such patients would only comprise those whose cervical cord has been damaged to an exceptionally large extent (i.e. where the transverse intramedullary rupture has destroyed axis cylinders and axially oriented small blood vessels within a large cross-sectional area of the cervical cord, followed by formation of a correspondingly large intramedullary scar).

It would seem therapeutically indefensible and economically unwise not to make use of the possibility for improving the degree of conductivity of traumatically compressed cervical spinal cord by exploiting an innate biological mechanism of the cord, for this can permit a higher rate and a higher level of rehabilitation of patients with spinal cord injuries to be attained. We therefore hope that this new therapeutic regime for patients with spinal injuries will soon gain wide interest and application.

The present therapeutic conception can meet the claim to be conservative to an even greater extent than the well-tried and efficacious programme of the International Medical Society of Paraplegia since it makes use of the innate *self-protecting* capacity for healing of the spinal cord tissue [18].

Part II
A New Approach to Improved Rehabilitation

7 Surgical Procedure for Cervicolordodesis

7.1 Introduction

In the treatment of peripheral entrapment neuropathies, where the conductivity of compressed and overstretched nerves must be restored, surgeons often prefer to change the course of the mechanically compromised nerve rather than to extirpate the offending lesion, which may be difficult to reach or even inaccessible. A well-known example of restoration of the conductivity of an imperiled nerve by changing its course is the transposition of the ulnar nerve from its normal topographical position to a new position in the elbow fold, where it is removed from the offending epicondyle so that it becomes slackened and is able to regain its conductivity.

Many spinal cord affections are likewise inaccessible to surgery. We therefore devised the operative technique which we term cervicolordodesis (CLD). This technique takes advantage of the innate telescoping mechanism of the spinal cord: by surgical fixation of the cervical spine in scarcely noticeable dorsiflexion, medullary tissue is made slack along the entire length of the cord. In its slackened state this tissue can escape potential harmful pressure of firm pathological matter outside of or within the cord, such as displaced bone, osseous outgrowth, tumour tissue and other unyielding organic matter. Neurological symptoms caused by local pressure on the spinal cord during its physiological tension (i.e. when the cervical spine is ventroflexed) are reduced or suppressed as soon as the cord becomes slack.

This novel idea of utilizing physiological relaxation of medullary tissue as a therapeutic technique widens the frontier of clinical neurology and brings hope of improvement to formerly inaccessible spinal cord disorders. The underlying principles of this technique are based on the following facts: As confirmed experimentally, in any part of the spinal cord tract where firm pathological matter exerts focal thrust on medullary tissue, axially oriented nerve fibres and capillaries in adjacent spinal cord pathways are invariably overstretched. According to a general neurophysiological principle, the respective nerve fibres cease to conduct as soon as they have been critically attenuated. However, they begin to propagate action potentials again (provided that they have not been damaged) when subdeleterious overstretching is eliminated, and they have thus regained their normal shape [7, 27, 35, 42].

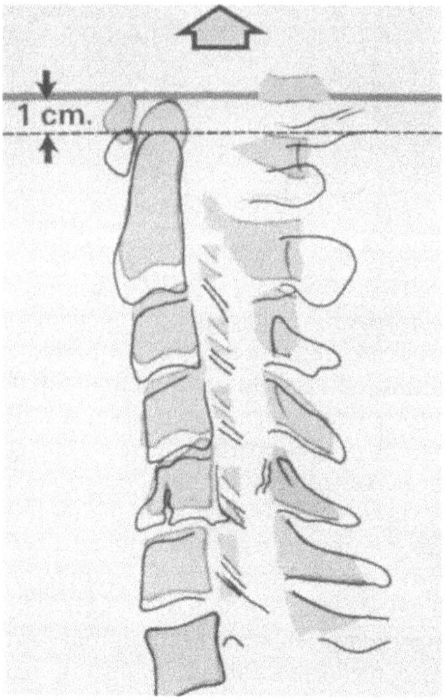

Fig. 17. Cervical spine of CLD pilot patient; lengthening of 10 mm had occurred during skull traction

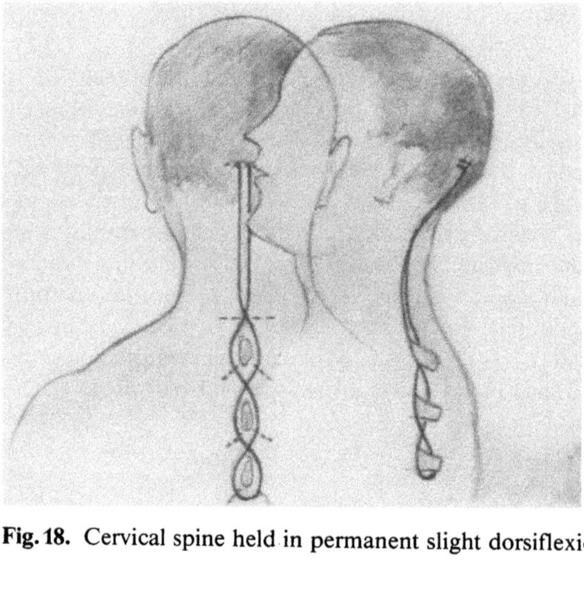

Fig. 18. Cervical spine held in permanent slight dorsiflexion by CLD

7.2 *Description of the Technique*

7.2.1 Topography

Figure 17 shows the cervical spine of our pilot CLD patient, whose case is reported on p.9; lengthening of 10 mm had occurred during skull traction. CLD holds the cervical spine in permanent slight dorsiflexion; the area involved extends from the lower part of the parietal bone to the upper thoracic processes (Fig. 18). Whereas the pressure caused by a rigid intramedullary body on neighbouring nerve fibres and blood vessels is exacerbated by ventroflexion of the neck, it is relieved by dorsiflexion, which relaxes the cervical cord (Figs. 19, 20). Surgically se-

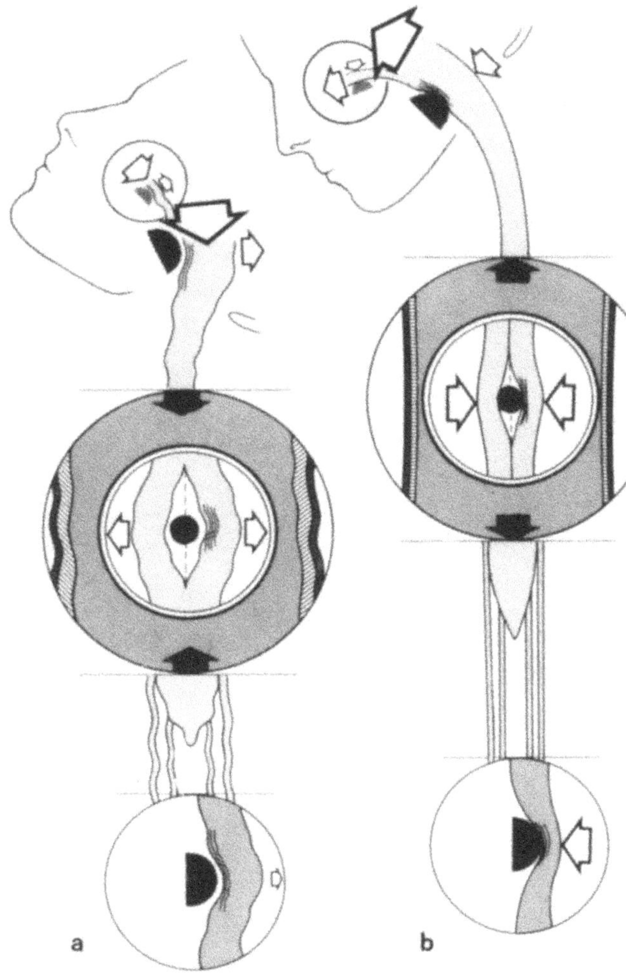

Fig. 19. Dorsiflexion of neck **(a)** relieves pressure caused by rigid intramedullary body on neighbouring nerve fibres, whereas ventroflexion **(b)** exacerbates it (cf. Fig. 20)

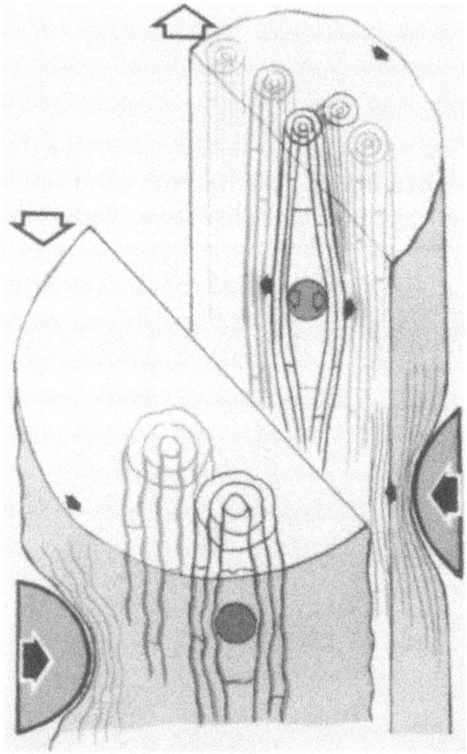

Fig. 20. Relaxation of cervical spinal cord *(lower)* relieves pressure of rigid intramedullary body on neighbouring nerve fibres, whereas stretching *(upper)* exacerbates it (cf. Fig. 19)

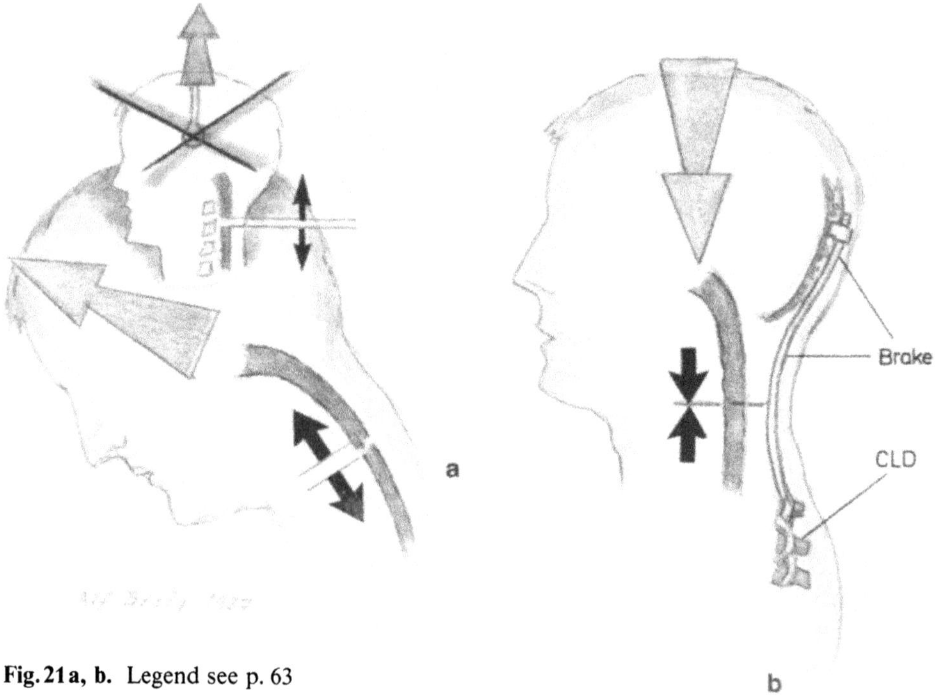

Fig. 21 a, b. Legend see p. 63

cured lordosis of the cervical spine (CLD) is also beneficial in the case of post-traumatic rupture of the cervical cord: as demonstrated in Fig. 21, both spinal ventroflexion and skull traction cause the surfaces of an intramedullary wound to retract, whilst spinal dorsiflexion closes the gap and thus encourages healing processes.

7.2.2 Equipment

The following items are required for performance of the CLD operation:

- CLD ribbon. This is a woven polyester ribbon consisting of polyethylene terephthalate and 0.04% titanium oxide (Trevira-Hochfest 730, Hoechst, Frankfurt, Federal Republic of Germany). The CLD ribbon can be sterilized several times, it fulfils the requirements of § 177.1630 Code Federal Regulation of the United States Food and Drug Administration. (In trials with implantation into sheep front legs for 170 days, CLD ribbon has proven histocompatible and has been found to respond to a continuous dynamic load by a 0.68% increase in length [26].)
- A small clamp, measuring 25 × 5 × 6 mm, used for securement of the CLD ribbon to the parietal bone (Fig. 22). (All instruments for the CLD procedure are manufacted by Aesculap-Werke, Tuttlingen, Federal Republic of Germany.)
- Two differently shaped applicators, as illustrated in Fig. 23, used to anchor the CLD ribbon under the interspinal ligament.
- An instrument designed for pulling the CLD ribbon through the neck muscles (Fig. 24).

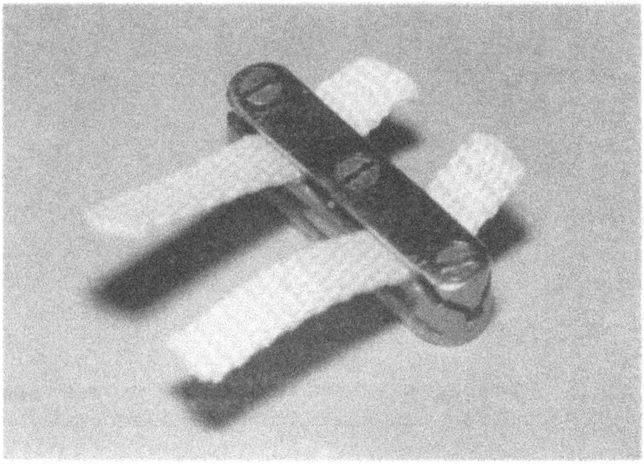

Fig. 22. Clamp for anchorage of the CLD ribbon in the parietal bone

◁ **Fig. 21.** Retraction **(a)** of surfaces of an intramedullary wound upon spinal ventroflexion and skull traction and closing of gap **(b)** upon dorsiflexion

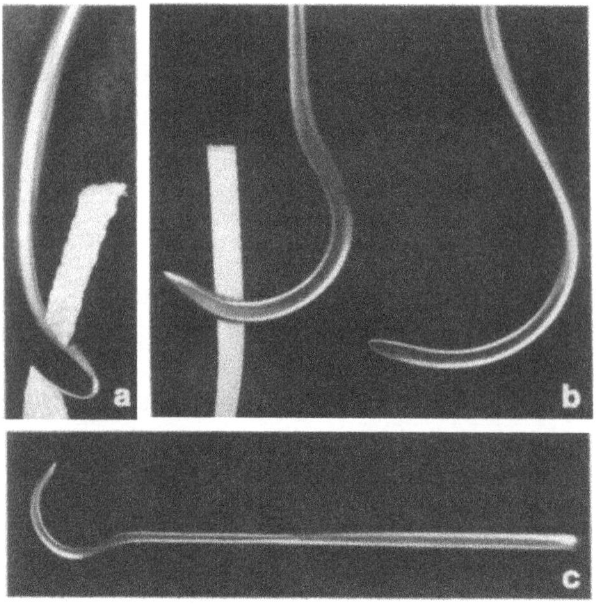

Fig. 23a–c. Applicators for CLD ribbon. **a** With a shorter curvature for anchoring the CLD ribbon transversely under the interspinal ligament caudal to the third thoracic spinous process. **b** With a wider curvature for anchoring the CLD ribbon diagonally under the interspinal ligament (cf. Fig. 18). **c** Total view of the applicator with its flat handle at 90° in relation to the sagitally oriented edge of its curved end

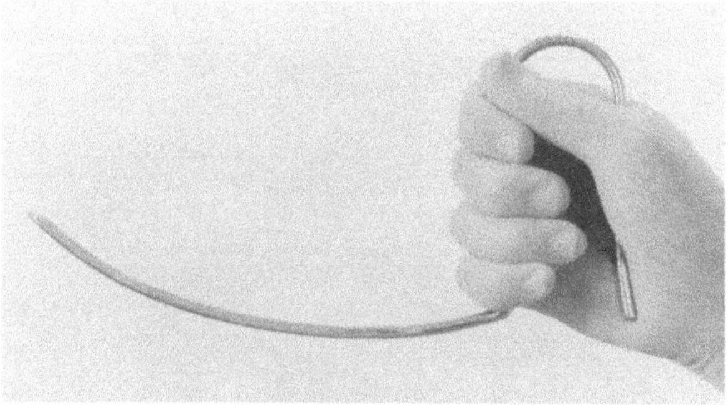

Fig. 24. Triangular instrument (gliding with its broad surface on the cervical spinous processes) for pulling the CLD ribbon through (underneath) neck muscles

7.2.3 Preliminary Measurements

Prior to CLD certain measurements must be made on the thickness of bone structures which are to serve as points of anchorage for various instruments used in the CLD immobilization/relaxation. These are:

- The depth of the parietal bone, a few millimetres above the transverse sinus of the dura mater, on conventional tomograms or CT images in three sagittal planes: one in the midline and the other two 12 mm on either side of and parallel to the midline. (Knowledge of the thickness of the parietal bone at these sites allows the length of the drill to be set so that it cannot damage the dura mater.)
- The anteroposterior width of the cervical canal at all levels on tomograms of the cervical spine in the CLD posture (where the length of the concave posterior aspect of the cervical canal is shortened by about 1.5 cm compared with its length in the erect posture).

CLD is contraindicated when the anteroposterior width of the cervical canal is less than 13 mm at any level, for this would mean that the cervical cord might be exposed to compression during the CLD procedure. While this is being assessed, the effect of maximum dorsiflexion of the cervical spine on the anteroposterior width of the cervical canal should also be investigated (provided that there are no pathological changes which render this posture contraindicated): CLD in, for example, a situation involving whiplash in which the cervical spine is forcibly bent backwards. Contrary to the conventional view we regard any stable deformity of the cervical spine/canal as acceptable with regard to CLD so long as it does not prevent effective relaxation of the spinal cord [16].

7.2.4 Performance of Operation

In CLD a small transverse groove just above the lambdoid suture is drilled mediosagitally in the parietal bone to allow the clamp (Fig. 22) to be cemented into it (Fig. 18). Starting with small skin incisions as points of entry, bilateral to the three uppermost thoracic processes, a 5-mm wide, non-elastic Trevira ribbon is anchored by a shoe-lacing technique, deep under the interspinous ligaments around the above-mentioned processes (Figs. 18, 19). Insertion of the ribbon and pulling it into place is a quick procedure which is made possible today by the use of a ribbon applicator, shown in Fig. 23. With the aid of another special instrument (Fig. 24) the now cranially directed ends of the CLD ribbon are then pulled through a deep sagittal tunnel in the neck muscles to the clamp in the parietal bone, where they are firmly fixed (Fig. 21). The length of the CLD ribbon is adjusted in situ so that it causes a sudden stop when the head and cervical spine are just about to leave the position in which relaxation of the spinal cord is guaranteed. After completion of CLD the patient is able to dorsiflex the head and cervical spine freely and to turn them sideways but is no longer able to bend them forwards (Fig. 21 b).

7.2.5 Spinal Stability: A Basic Prerequisite

In patients who have sustained a spinal cord injury reliable stability of the cervical spine must have been reestablished by orthopaedic-surgical measures before CLD can be applied. Also in chronically disabled persons the spine must be perfectly stable to allow therapeutic CLD relaxation of the cervical spinal cord. With its further perfection, magnetic resonance imaging will probably soon contribute valuable preoperative criteria for selection of patients for CLD treatment, both among those with acute spinal cord injury and among those with chronic spinal cord disorders.

Isometric exercises for the neck muscles are recommended to all patients who have undergone CLD.

7.3 Case Report

Table 11 reproduces a questionnaire filled out in 1987 by a man aged 57 years who 6 years previously had undergone CLD because of incapacitating neurological symptoms of cervical myelopathy. This patient, whose experiences confirm that a locked neck causes only slight inconvenience, was chosen for demonstration purposes only because he was easiest to get in touch with. In his case, the regression of the neurological signs and symptoms of cervical myelopathy had been rather slow compared with that in patients in a previous series who showed immediate improvement [7].

Photographs of this patient are presented in Figs. 25-27. As is apparent from Fig. 25, the patient has regained full control of balance since the CLD operation, and he is by no means hampered by the inability to bend his neck forward to no more than its upright posture.

Table 11. Questionnaire filled out by a 57-year-old patient after undergoing CLD operation

Please answer following questions about CLD:	Yes	No	Hours	Days	Months
Has it been troublesome to get accustomed to limited neck bending?		+			
How long did it take to get accustomed to a "locked neck"?			+		
Are you satisfied with the results?	+				
Do you consider the price paid by limited neck bending reasonable in relation to the advantages gained?	+				
Do you feel disabled?		+			
Would you recommend CLD to other persons disabled by the same ailment as your previous one?	+				

Table 11 *(continued)*

Do persons in your environment react?	Yes	No	Often	Seldom
Has anybody noticed that you have an abnormal posture?		Never		
Has anybody asked you about your reduced ability to bend your neck forward?		Never		
Are you personally often reminded of your limited ability to flex your neck?		Never		

Which of the daily movements/ occupations listed below do you today grade as:	Normal (easy)	Difficult	Impossible	Special disturbing circumstances
Dressing yourself	+			
Fastening buttons			+[a]	Reduced sensibility in fingers
Putting on shoes	+			
Tying shoelaces		+[a]		
Eating from a plate at table	+			
Descending steps		+[b]		Slow because of difficulty in seeing steps
Writing at a desk	+	to +[a]		
Washing different parts of the body	+			Cannot reach my back
Watching television	+			
Picking up objects from the floor	+			
Changing your position in bed	+			
Orientation in traffic	+			
Driving a car	+			
Running		+[a]		Right leg heavy

[a] Difficulties in writing, buttoning and running are not caused by CLD but are residual symptoms of myelopathy/radiculopathy (see case report on p. 71).
[b] Direct CLD sequelae: virtually only descending of stairs has become more difficult.

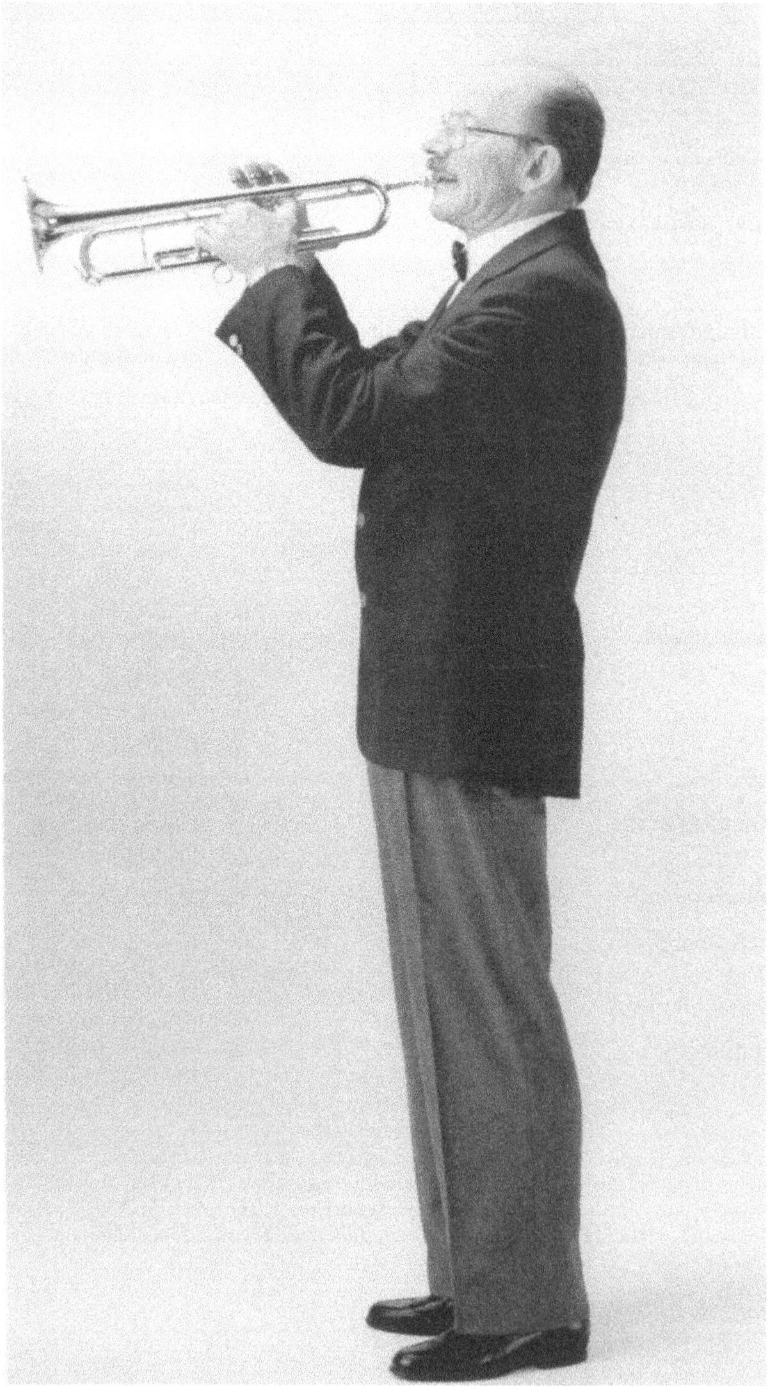

Fig. 25. The patient who filled out the questionnaire in Table 11, 6 years after a CLD operation. Full control of legs has been regained

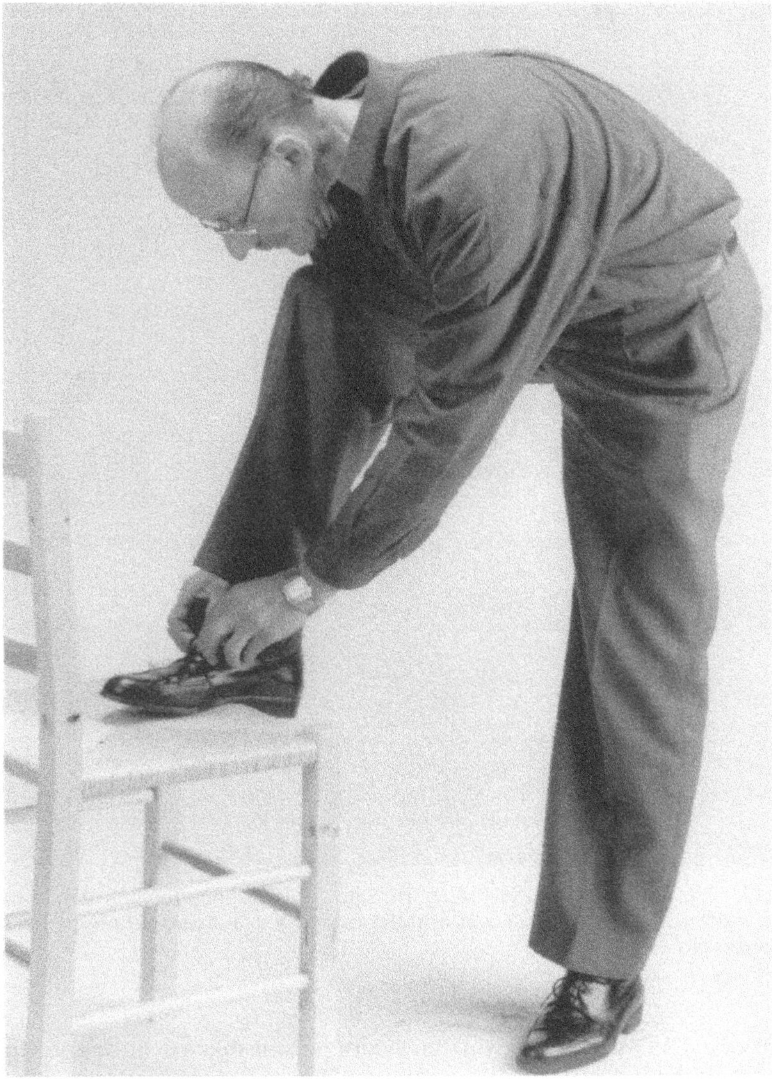

Fig. 26. The same patient as in Fig. 25. The greater part of the vertebral column has retained full mobility

Figure 26 shows that the greatest part of the vertebral column of this man with a CLD-locked neck has retained full mobility; when he bends forward to tie his shoelaces, the contour of his posterior neckline remains perfectly straight (indicating that the cervical column itself has retained its slightly dorsiflexed posture). The dorsal and lumbar columns are, however, bent forward in a harmonious arch, so that the inability of the patient to bend his head forward is obviously largely compensated. When one looks at the relatively marked ventroflexion of the thoracic and lumbar spine of this man, one may perhaps wonder whether the spinal

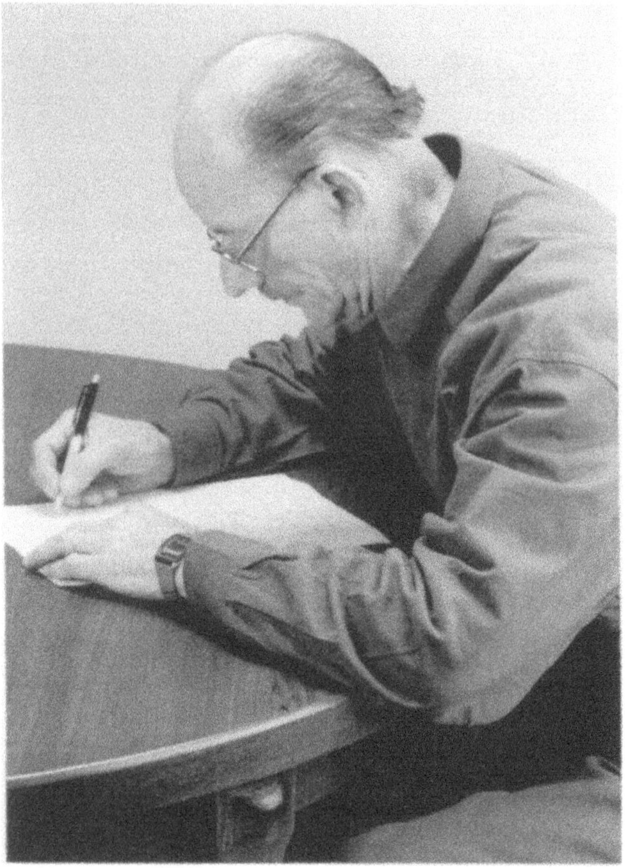

Fig. 27. The same patient as in Fig. 25. In spite of his inability to ventroflex the head further than is shown here, writing and most other everyday activities are unimpeded by the CLD-locked neck

cord of a CLD-treated person can really remain relaxed during maximal ventroflexion of the rest of the spinal column. However, as shown above, since the cervical canal shortens most of all sections of the spinal canal during dorsiflexion of the spinal column and therefore produces the greatest reserve of relaxed dura and cord, even a minor degree of shortening of the cervical canal (as that established by CLD) will suffice to keep the spinal cord perfectly relaxed along its entire length. The statement by the patient described above that he is essentially unimpeded by his CLD-locked neck when writing at his desk would seem to be fully confirmed by Fig. 27. As indicated by the straight posterior contour of his neck, it would seem likely that he has bent his neck forward as far as possible, i.e. until the CLD brake has come into action. Nevertheless, from his relaxed and natural posture while writing, probably no one would suspect that his neck is permanently locked, and that he cannot ventroflex his head more than to the posture seen in the photograph.

Clinical Record

- Neurological History. Early in 1980 the patient complained of radiating pain and paraesthesia in the neck and arms and of numbness in the right thumb. He had increasing difficulty in walking and was forced to drag and circumduct the right leg. He was troubled by increasing urinary incontinence.
- Neurological Findings. Paraesthesia in the legs with diminished vibratory sensation. Perception of touch reduced most on posterior aspect of thorax. Segmental motor deficit and fasciculations predominantly in the right arm and leg. Bilateral hyporeflexia of biceps muscles. Electromyogram: bilateral C-5 degeneration. Hyperreflexia in both legs, patellar clonus, and Babinski's sign positive on right side.
- Radiographic Examination. Myelography and tomography showed large protrusions at the level C-4/C-5 with a filling defect of the subarachnoid space at the same level.
- Operation (by M. Renard, 6 March 1981, Hôpital St. Julien, Nancy, France). Removal of the vertebral bodies of C-4 and C-5, replaced by iliac transplant. Postoperative course uneventful. After 4-5 months, persistent signs of tetraspasticity. One week prior to reoperation: slow, extremely spastic gait with circumduction of right leg, had to pause every 6-8 m.
- Reoperation (by A. Breig and M. Renard, 2 July 1981, Hôpital St. Julien, Nancy, France). CLD (for technique, see p. 65). A few days after surgery, slight discharge from region of uppermost dorsal spinous process, stopped after compression bandage. 8 September 1981: still exaggerated reflexes and neck pain, radiating to arms and hands. 8 March 1982: considerably improved gait. Had participated in a 10-day excursion to Upper Volta with walks in the bush. 17 April 1982; single puncture with sterile fluid collection at level of CLD prosthesis. 10 October 1986: normalized deep sensibility. No longer any urethral sphincter trouble. Had full control of legs: could play the trumpet whilst parading in the street. However, he continued to have neck pain and reduced sensibility in the fingers, especially those of the right hand. (Note: persistent compression of cervical nerve roots could have been relieved by surgical widening of the intervertebral foramina.)

8 Therapeutic Breadth of Surgically Secured Spinal Cord Relaxation

Clinical experience with CLD over several years has confirmed that surgically secured slackening of the spinal cord can remove obstacles to the transmission of impulses along medullary pathways and can relieve neurological deficit, whether elicited by an offending lesion in the immediate vicinity of the cervical cord or by a lesion within its tissue. Besides slackening of overstretched nerve fibres, spinal cord relaxation also contributes to restoration of cord conductivity by increasing the oxygenation of medullary tissue, since it causes widening of the lumina of overstretched/constricted small blood vessels [37]; improved conductivity can be traced and followed by recording of evoked potentials.

Concerning the rapidity of neurological improvement after CLD, the conductivity of blocked spinal pathways returns often strikingly quickly when focal pressure of unyielding firm lesions on the spinal cord has been relieved; early clinical restoration of sensation, motor ability and bladder control seems to be the rule rather than the exception.

With regard to the biomechanical extent of its therapeutic efficacy, CLD has proven to enhance the conductivity of medullary pathways along the whole length of the spinal cord in most pathological conditions, when the size of the lesion encroaching on the spinal canal or distending the cord from inside is not too large to permit the relaxed cord tissue to pass beneath it without being exposed to pressure. In practice, the final effect of CLD is therefore equivalent to that of extirpation of the respective lesion.

In the chronically disabling cord disorders that are now amenable to treatment, focal pressure of unyielding extra- and intramedullary lesions on the spinal cord (triggering the neurological symptoms in question) is invariably generated whenever the spinal cord is elastically stretched. Stretching of the spinal cord, and hence the triggering of symptoms, begins almost exactly when the patient's cervical spine is just on the verge of being ventroflexed, and the spinal cord is thus undergoing physiological elastic tension. The basic view that cord stretching is the symptom-producing mechanism was coincidentally demonstrated in some patients who, because of initial insufficiency of the CLD technique, could again bend their necks increasingly far forward and whose neurological conditions therefore relapsed; after reoperation with the improved CLD technique now available the neurological symptoms again disappeared and were permanently relieved [7, 12, 13].

This insight today provides a rationale for surgical action and an effective means of reducing even those signs and symptoms of impeded conductivity and neurological deficit whose cause has hitherto been beyond therapeutic reach. On this basis it is now possible to have a more precise idea of the therapeutic breadth of the CLD procedure.

The category of chronically disabling cord disorders whose symptoms can now be mitigated or even eliminated includes fresh and chronic sequelae of traumatic spinal cord injury, cervical myelopathy, multiple sclerosis with foci predominantly in the cervical spinal cord, intramedullary cysts and haemangioma [7, 11, 20]. Clinical records of several patients suffering from sequelae of spinal cord injury (including our pilot patient with a fresh spinal cord injury referred to on p.9) shows that one of the first effects of CLD-induced cord relaxation is frequently the alleviation of urinary incontinence. Even if no further symptoms than this could be relieved in these patients, CLD would certainly be fully justified, since elimination of incontinence can mean restoration of human dignity and can give these patients a higher quality of life.

Due to hesitancy traditionally on the part of referring physicians it has been possible thus far to treat only a relatively small number of patients with the CLD procedure. For this reason we do not yet have at our disposal a sufficiently wide set of data for scientific evaluation of the overall therapeutic potential of CLD in the aforementioned disorders. However, the clinical observations reported here demonstrate that neurological functions have improved strikingly in patients with these types of neurological disorders, of different pathogenetic origins. It therefore seems probable that this measure will gain widespread application by virtue of its remarkably broad therapeutic range.

8.1 Research on Indications for CLD in Patients with Chronic Spinal Cord Disorders

Readers seeking more detailed information about the nature of spinal cord lesions that cause neurological disability, and that can potentially be reduced, or even totally ameliorated, by surgically secured relaxation of the spinal cord are referred to p.250 of the 1978 monograph by the present author [7]; here there are listed all presently known disorders of the brain stem, spinal cord and nerve roots which may be treated by CLD. For the majority of cord lesions enumerated here we have proven the occurrence of surgically secured slackening of medullary tissue in at least some patients and have thereby confirmed that this measure leads to restoration of neurological functions. However, in two or three of the listed disorders, e.g. amyotrophic lateral sclerosis (ALS), the probable beneficial effects of CLD could, at the time of that writing, only be speculated upon on the basis of hypotheses derived from analyses of the experimental behaviour of medullary tissue.

One critic of our procedures, who stated that he had found no convincing evidence for their potential benefit, complained that "the clinical value of the operations is not systematically documented in a larger control series of patients" [62]. This critic was evidently unaware, however, that the data presented in the 1978 monograph comprised only preliminary results of basic research into a growing field, the boundaries of which can only gradually be delineated. Any reader of the present work cannot but conclude from our elaborate case reports that all patients operated on by the CLD method have improved; he will also note that the course and rate of their improvement is referred to in detail. No failures have been excluded from publication. It is clear that, compaired with those submitted to nonspecific conventional neurosurgical methods, patients treated with the new biological CLD procedure have obviously superior chances of neurological improvement.

The inclusion of ALS in the above list of disorders suitable for CLD treatment is motivated by the desire to encourage attempts at testing the value of medullary slackening in this serious condition. In a disorder with such alarming symptoms as those in ALS, it would seem especially inappropriate to delay the simple surgical measure of keeping the neck fixed in slight dorsiflexion whilst awaiting, for example, the approval of an ethics committee. When, therefore, a woman in her fifties was admitted to a hospital in Nancy, France, some years ago, suffering from ALS and cervical myelopathy, we followed the above programme and performed the CLD operation. Within a few days not only was her spasticity diminished and urinary incontinence reduced, but her swallowing was also clearly facilitated. Some weeks after this operation we were informed that this patient continued to improve; however, we subsequently learned that she had died some months later after having been treated at a physiotherapy institution with - among other measures - forcible forward bending of her neck (!). This case justifies pursuit of the therapeutic possiblities which CLD offers also in patients with relatively rare conditions such as ALS. Recent research on ALS has focused on the possible role of enzymatic disturbances. However, analogously to the case of multiple sclerosis, where, irrespective of the presumed activity of allergenic and other factors, CLD relaxation of the affected cord tissue has proved to alleviate urinary incontinence and sensory and motor disturbances, in ALS beneficial neurological effects of CLD alone are within the range of possibility.

In view of our clinical observations of the beneficial effects of CLD in spinal cord disorders, there is every reason to continue to explore the degree of effectiveness of this potent new therapeutic tool in various chronic cord disorders and to apply it accordingly, with no other restrictions than clear clinical contraindications.

Regarding the indications for treatment of, for example, chronic post-traumatic sequelae of spinal cord injury and multiple sclerosis, it is now possible to predict the extent of CLD restoration of preserved but concealed neurological functions by examining them preoperatively with the use of evoked potentials [39, 55, 56].

9 Summary of Part II

9.1 Therapeutic Skull Traction: A Failed Experiment

As is apparent from the results of the investigations reported here, therapeutic skull traction can be regarded as a neurobiological experiment which, instead of protecting traumatized cervical cord, has in reality exposed it to varying degrees of non-physiological stretching and has thus kept neurological improvement at a lower level than would have been made possible by the use of methods for cord relaxation. With this insight it would seem appropriate to ask whether biomechanically induced intramedullary overstretching may play a similarly adverse role in other complex situations, where some relevant factors are not yet fully elucidated, for example, in trials to restore the conductivity of the severed cord by growth-inducing hormones, gene technologically enhanced reparative growth or various types of grafts.

A field in which this question arises is that of regeneration after spinal cord injury. As is generally well known, Ramon y Cajal [53] showed that cut axis cylinders in a severed spinal cord react by outgrowth of sprouts with growth cones, a sign that they are fully prepared to make regenerative contact with their torn-off end. After about 2 weeks, however, this clear initial tendency to healing is unexpectedly inhibited. Ramon y Cajal, who coined the term "autotomy" for this puzzling degeneration, had no explanation for it, nor have so far even modern neurobiologists. In a joint study on the nature of the autodestructive forces following compressive spinal cord injury, we came to the conclusion that all available indications today point to the fact that, when transverse rupturing of the spinal cord has occurred, it is the physiological elastic stretching of the cord that causes the distal intramedullary wound surface to retract from its proximal counterpart, from which sprouts are growing out (Fig. 6), so that despite the presence of growth hormones and other neurobiologically active substances they finally dwindle; moreover, the sprouts are probably too feeble to withstand the forcible stretching of the medullary tissue following spinal ventroflexion.

We have often had the disappointing experience that readers are not entirely convinced by written reports on the adverse effects of biomechanical stretching of the cord on the constituent elements of the medullary tissue. This points to the need for direct visual demonstration of the retraction of the medullary wound surfaces from each other in a transected cervical cord, for example, in a fresh human cadaver. It is obvious that only direct observation of the forcible way in which the intramedullary wound surfaces are drawn apart when the cervical spine is ventroflexed (a phenomenon that occurs in the same way in the severed cord of all experimental vertebrates) can be fully convincing that this powerful force is bound to destroy either the sprouts themselves or the tissue fibres along which sprouts could grow out and reach their cut-off distal ends or other targets.

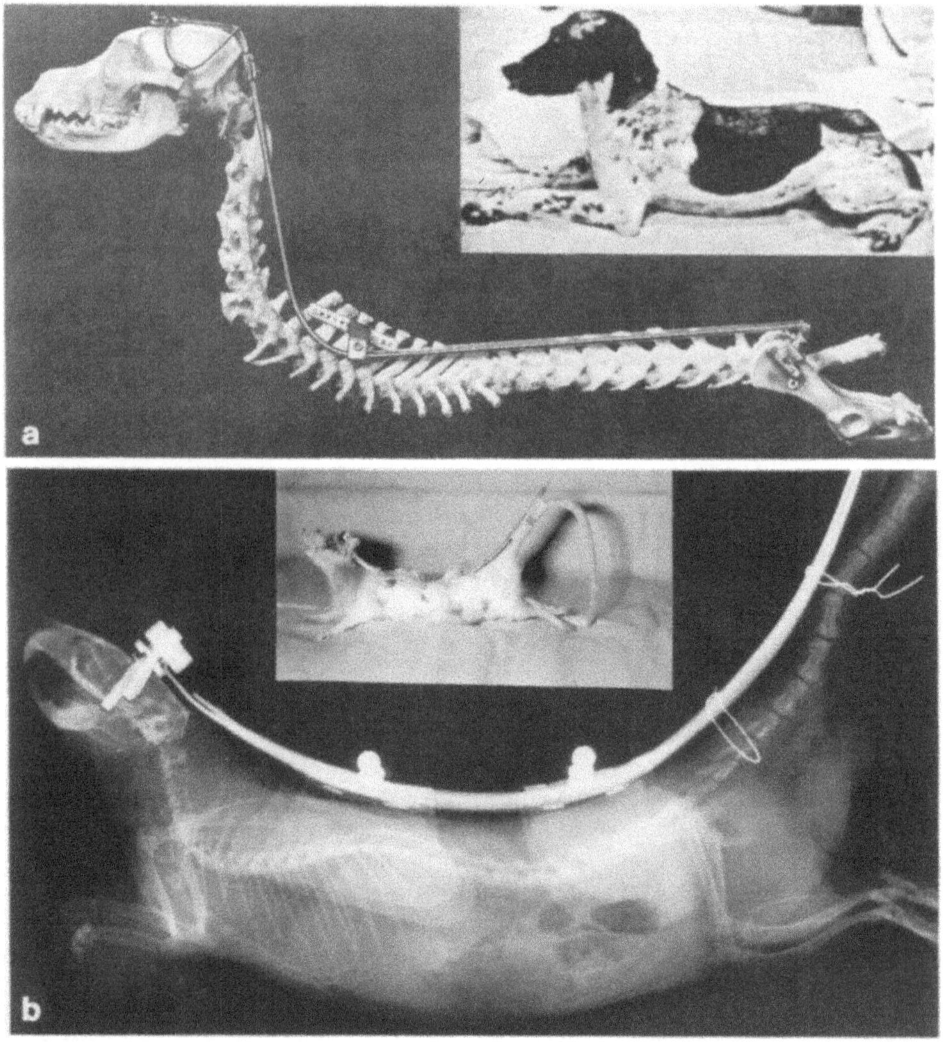

Fig. 28 a, b. Devices for thorough immobilization of the vertebrate spinal column with a dorsiflexed cervical spine. **a** Device for the dog ("Rotterdam apparatus") constructed in collaboration with engineers at the Central Research Workshop, Erasmus University, Rotterdam, Netherlands [17, 18]. **b** Device for the rat (Breig - rat cord relaxation frame). Technique for surgical fixation of the head piece has been worked out (in about twelve rats with an average weight of 220 g) in collaboration with Dr. Miyako Osawa (Department of Orthopaedic Surgery, Kanazawa University, Japan) at the Department of Neurobiology, University of Gothenburg, Sweden, 1985

Ramon y Cajal pointed out already long before our experiments that, after severance of the spinal cord, retraction of medullary axis cylinders is in many respects reminiscent of retraction of the stumps of a cut peripheral nerve. With knowledge of the biomechanics of the spinal cord the idea should have lain near at hand to test the well-tried technique - which in surgery of the cut peripheral nerve has long proven to give good functional results - of relaxing the medullary nerve cable and keeping its wound surfaces in prolonged close and tension-free contact until biological healing has occurred.

Experimental proof was obtained in a hemisected dog that the adverse effects of the deleterious stretching mechanism of the spinal cord on its own tissue can be successfully counteracted by applying a technique to the spinal cord, essentially similar to that used in surgical restoration of the conductivity of severed peripheral nerves. Six weeks after total immobilization of the dog's spine in dorsiflexion (and thereby with close, tension-free contact of the intramedullary wound surfaces) a small number of nerve fibres had regenerated and bridged the former wound cleft [17, 18]. To confirm the validity of this regeneration mechanism in a larger number of animals we have recently developed an immobilization harness for rats (Fig. 28). Owing to extrinsic circumstances, so far only a single rat has been kept anaesthetized and immobilized for 7 days with a dorsiflexed spine, after which this experiment was discontinued; a new form of anaesthesia for the rat, which we have developed for this purpose, has opened promising prospects [22, 60]. (Stumps of transected rat spinal cord show already after 1 week a clear tendency to coalesce when telescoped through dorsiflexion of the spine; see Fig. 29.)

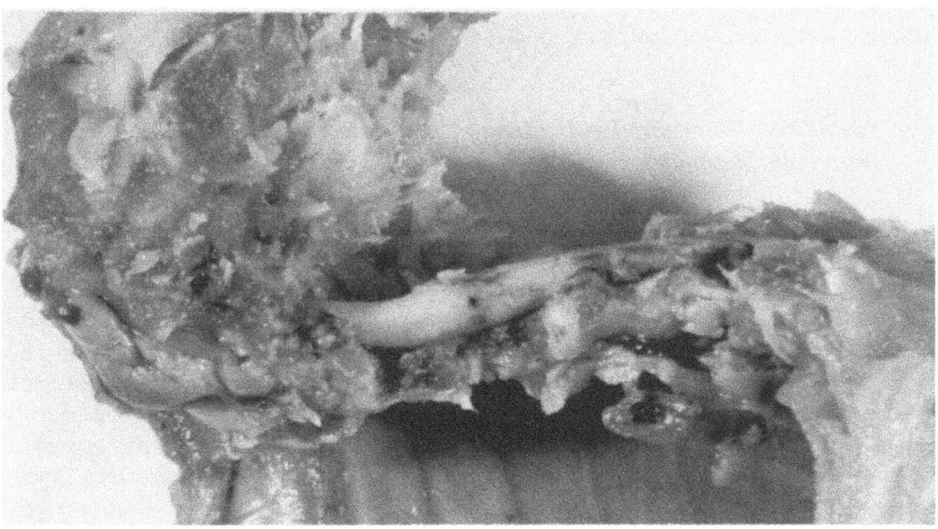

Fig. 29. Healing support of severed spinal cord. Coalesced stumps of transected rat thoracic cord (at T-4) in situ 6 days after tension-free apposition (through cord telescoping/relaxation) secured by total immobilization of the vertebral column (head-spine-tail) in dorsiflexion. The rat was kept under permanent 80% nitrous oxide anaesthesia [60] (cf. Fig. 28 **b**) and fixed by formaldehyde perfusion through the cardiac route. Parts of bones and tissues are left in place to show marked degree of cervical dorsiflexion *(upper left)*. For extraneous reasons, the experiment was terminated prematurely and the originally planned histological examination (using tracers) was not carried out. The striking degree of smooth restitution of the surface of the transected cord by long-term apposition of its relaxed stumps would seem to justify a thorough investigation of the possible reorganizing potential of this measure

With the aim of curing traumatic defects in the spinal cord, many neurobiologists are today engaged in research which seeks potent biological agents for stimulating the regeneration of medullary tissue [1, 51]. One of the current ideas in this area involves transplanting embryonic medullary tissue or injecting cultured multivalent nerve cells into the damaged part of the spinal cord. It seems likely, however, that newly formed medullary tissue from any source needs an appropriate period of time to become rooted in neighbouring organized medullary tissue; it also seems probable that, as in the healing of any other traumatized tissue in the human body, the damaged part of the spinal cord needs to be totally immobilized during the phase of its artificially stimulated regeneration. Thus, even if the endeavours of researchers throughout the world in the field of spinal cord injury finally prove successful, there is still a *final biomechanical hurdle* that can most probably be overcome only by total immobilization of the spinal cord in surgically secured relaxation for a period of time which is yet unknown.

From the above observations it may be concluded that the biomechanics of the pons-cord tissue tract generates autoaggressive forces against regeneration of medullary tissue. With elucidation of this phenomenon, the factor that has hitherto prevented effective therapeutic measures against paraplegia seems to have been identified.

The only practicable preventive measure today against biomechanical autoaggression of traumatized medullary tissue is surgical uncoupling of the ventroflexion mechanism of the cervical spine and fixation of this part of the spine in slight, scarcely noticeable physiological dorsiflexion.

9.2 Innate Self-Protecting Relaxation for Restoring Conductivity in Damaged Medullary Tissue

Today an innate self-protecting relaxation mechanism of the spinal cord can be utilized to protect traumatically thinned cervical cord tissue from further deleterious stretching. The patient's cervical spine needs to be only slightly dorsiflexed, whereupon the spinal cord becomes slack along its entire length (as any rope slackens when its ends are approximated to each other). To obtain room in the now shortened spinal canal the soft medullary tissue of the spinal cord telescopes into undulating folds. Traumatically overstretched nerve fibres and small blood vessels thus become effectively relaxed and can regain their conductivity/conveyability; internal surfaces of transverse medullary ruptures are brought into close, tension-free apposition. Even if no viable regeneration is achieved, this measure reduces the amount of intramedullary haemorrhage and scar formation, thus ensuring improved conductivity of nerve fibres in neighbouring pathways which would otherwise have been jeopardized by the multilateral thrust of a potential scar. To prevent impairment of neurological functions by sequelae of a spinal cord injury deleterious stretching of the spinal cord must obviously be counteracted by rendering it permanently impossible to flex the cervical spine forward. This can be done by the CLD operation.

In a number of patients who were disabled after a cervical cord injury, and whose neurological performances considerably improved after surgically secured spinal cord relaxation (CLD), the respective functions again quickly deteriorated when (because of technical mishaps) their slackened medullary tissue again came under increased tension, resulting in relapse of the preoperative neurological deficit. The deficit again disappeared, however, shortly after the spinal cord had been made slack by an improved technique.

In tetraplegic patients who have been rehabilitated to a wheelchair existence, the tissue of the cervical cord is nevertheless still exposed to chronic pressure of intramedullary scars: every time the head and neck are bent forwards the scars in the cervical cord press on nerve fibres in undamaged neighbouring long spinal pathways. As a result the potential conductivity of these nerve fibres is effectively suppressed as long as they are intermittently overstretched by exertion of thrust upon them by the respective scars. If, however, the cervical cord of these disabled persons had been relaxed by permanent slight extension of the cervical spine, the intramedullary scars in question would no longer be capable of pressing on and thus stretching nerve fibres in the surrounding normal pathways; the degree of neurological disability in these persons would therefore be lower. At present, it cannot be predicted which suppressed (dormant) neurological functions may be awakened in tetraplegic patients by permanent relaxation of the cervical cord. Electrical epidural stimulation and recording of evoked potentials might offer a means of determining which neurological functions can either be awakened or improved by CLD. To obtain reliable results, dormant conductivity of the cord should be tested in its relaxed state.

With the present insight into the nature and extent of damage to medullary tissue caused by traumatic cord compression it is evident that the routine rehabilitation methods practised today are unsatisfactory. The disturbing effects of these lesions can today be attenuated by permanent relaxation of the cervical spinal cord. However successful, any rehabilitation of persons with spinal injuries must therefore be regarded today as still imperfect as long as the self-protecting biological relaxation of the spinal cord has not been utilized for optimum restoration of even small concealed residua of its former conductivity.

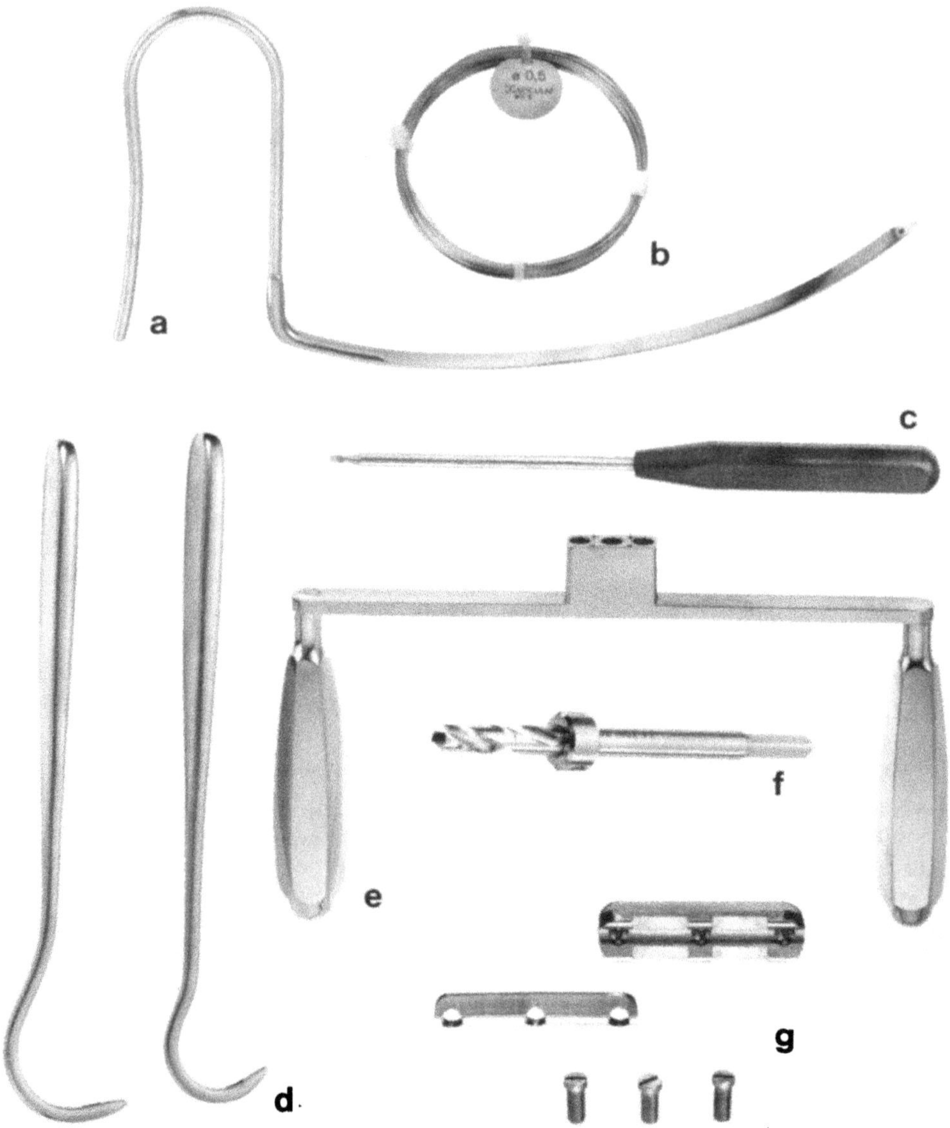

Fig. 30 a–g. Complete assembly of CLD instruments (the portrayed instruments are samples) manufactured and distributed by Aesculap-Werke AG, Tuttlingen, Federal Republic of Germany. **a** Triangular clamp for axial transfixation of CLD ribbon in neck muscles. **b** Wire, weak, Ø 0.5 mm, Aesculap-Art. No. KY 5 S. **c** Screwdriver for implant screws. **d** Instruments for pulling CLD ribbon across (underneath) interspinous ligaments. **e** Templet with handles for drilling groove for implant in parietal bone. **f** Drill, fitting into holes of templet, equipped with depth stop. **g** Implant (lock) for fixation of CLD ribbon

Head-Neck Posture After Completed CLD Operation

In our experience, the degree of dorsiflexion of the head and cervical spine required for relaxation of the spinal cord will be adequate when a line drawn through the orbitale (an anthropometric landmark representing the lowermost point on the inferior margin of the orbit) and the auditory foramen forms an angle of 10°-15° with the horizontal line. With the patient's head in this position, we have hitherto measured the distance from the jugular notch to the chin (i.e. the lower border of the mandible) with a ruler. We have then cut a piece of wood to the size of the distance between the jugular notch and the chin. With the patient in the prone position on the operating table, about to undergo CLD, we have then held this marker in place between the patient's chin and the sternum, thereby reproducing the degree of dorsiflexion of his head and cervical spine necessary to relax the spinal cord. To replace this relatively primitive procedure - which has to be used for the time being - by a more convenient method, we have long planned a measuring instrument (made of plastic or aluminium) for preoperative determination of the degree of dorsiflexion of the cervical spine. The lower end of this instrument should rest on the jugular notch of the sternum. To its upper end, two differently shaped measuring tips can be attached: one to establish the distance from the notch to the lower border of the mandible (*right* in the figure), the other for establishing the distance to the lower edge of the upper incisor teeth (*left*). The latter measure is probably more reliable, since in this case there are no interjacent soft tissues cranially that can interfere with accurate measuring.

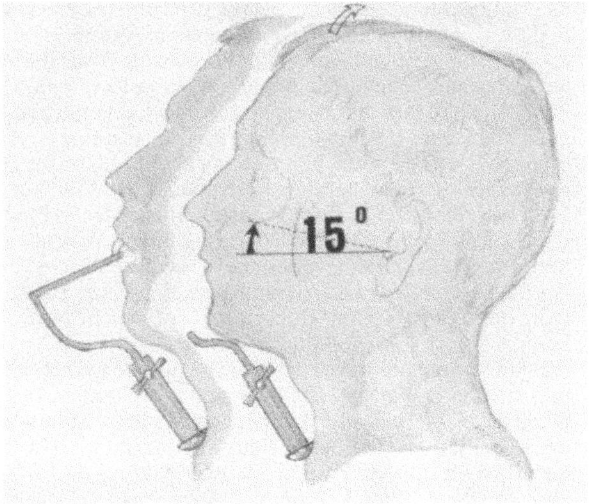

Fig. 31. Head extension calibrator, a device projected for preoperative determination of the head and neck posture to be attained on completion of the CLD operation

10 References

1. Aguayo AJ (1985) Axonal regeneration from injured neurons in central nervous system. In: Cotman CW (ed) Synaptic plasticity. Guilford, London, pp 457-484
2. Allen AR (1911) Surgery of experimental lesion of spinal cord equivalent to crush injury of fracture dislocation of spinal column. JAMA Sept 9, 878-880
3. Bedbrook GM (1979) Spinal injuries with tetraplegia and paraplegia. J Bone Joint Surg (Br) 61B: 267-284
4. Bedbrook GM (ed) (1981) The care and management of spinal cord injuries. Springer, Berlin Heidelberg New York
5. Böhler J (1982) Anterior stabilization for acute fractures and non-unions of the dens. J Bone Joint Surg (Am) 64A: 18-27
6. Breig A (1960) Biomechanics of the central nervous system. Almqvist and Wiksell, Stockholm; Year Book, Chicago
7. Breig A (1978) Adverse mechanical tension in the central nervous system. An analysis of cause and effect. Relief by functional neurosurgery. Almqvist and Wiksell, Stockholm; Wiley, New York
8. Breig A (1981) Spinal cord injury reduction and spinal stabilization: intramedullary stresses in compressive spinal cord injury; therapeutic countermeasures by exploiting spinal cord relaxation-telescoping. Lecture at NATO ASI in spinal cord injury rehabilitation engineering, Stoke Mandeville Hospital, Aylesbury, England, 13 May 1981
9. Breig A (1983) Biomechanical approach to restore dormant neurological functions in tetra- or paraplegic patients using surgery to relax the traumatized cord. Paper read at Annual International Medical Society of Paraplegia Meeting, Aylesbury, 18-20 May 1983
10. Breig A (1983) Biomechanical approach to restore dormant neurological functions in tetra- or paraplegic patients using surgery to relax the traumatized cord. 35th Meeting Scandinavian Neurosurgical Society, Hanasaari, Espöö, Finland, 1-4 June 1983
11. Breig A (1983) Post-traumatic syringomyelia. Pathogenesis. Paper read at Meeting, Postgraduate Centre, National Spinal Injuries Institute, Aylesbury, 18 July 1983
12. Breig A (1984) Surgical biomechanical procedure for restoration of neurological functions after traumatic para- and tetraplegia. (In German.) In: Hohmann D, Kügelgen B, Liebig K, Schirmer M (eds) Lendenwirbelsäulenerkrankungen mit Beteiligung des Nervensystems. Springer, Berlin Heidelberg New York
13. Breig A (1984) Biomechanisches Verfahren zur Wiederherstellung neurologischer Ausfälle bei tetraplegischen und paraplegischen Patienten mittels operativer Entspannung des traumatisierten Rückenmarks. Fortschr Neurol Psychiatr 52: 2-5
14. Breig A (1984) Spinal cord injury. Biotechnological repair of the ruptured cord in spinal injury and mitigation of its chronic sequelae: a compendium. Expanded version of data presented at Stoke Mandeville Hospital, Aylesbury, 18 July 1984
15. Breig A (1984) Failure of biomechanical adaptation mechanism of spinal cord in compressive injury. Neurological signs and symptoms. (In German.) Paper read at German-Greek symposium on paraplegia, Bad Wildungen, FRG, 2 Sept 1984
16. Breig A (1985) The CLD method. Paper read at Austrian AO seminar, Salzburg, 2 Oct 1985
17. Breig A, Renard M (1980) Effects of surgically secured spinal cord relaxation (telescoping) on healing process in hemisected canine lumbar spinal cords. A preliminary report. Transections of 1st international symposium on spinal cord reconstruction, Las Vegas, 7-10 January 1980

18. Breig A, Renard M, Stefanko S, Renard C (1982) Healing of the severed spinal cord by biomechanical relaxation and surgical immobilization. Anat Clin 4: 167-181
19. Breig A, Renard M (1982) Cervicolordodesis and its prospective therapeutic capacity in treatment of acute and chronic compressive spinal cord injury. (Studies in model wounds in experimental animals and in human cadavers.) Submitted to Paraplegia
20. Breig A, Troup JDG (1984) Focal intramedullary tension in patients with cord lesions and its surgical relief by spinal cord relaxation. Lancet I, March 31: 739-740
21. Breig A, Renard M (1986) Healing of spinal cord injury by biomechanical activation of growth of ruptured medullary tissue. In: Ghista DN (ed) Spinal cord injury medical engineering. Thomas, Springfield
22. Breig A, Renard M, Renard C (1987) New methods of neurological surgery for promoting biological repair of mechanically damaged spinal cord. Submitted to Bull Assoc Anat (Nancy)
23. Cloward RB (1973) Skull traction for cervical spine injury: should it be abandoned? JAMA 226: 1008
24. Cloward RB (1980) Acute cervical spine injuries. CIBA Symposia 32: 1
25. Colachis SC, Strohm BR (1966) Effect of duration of intermittent cervical traction on vertebral separation. Arch Phys Med 46: 820
26. Contzen H (1985) Materialtechnische Voraussetzungen und biologische Grundlagen für den alloplastischen Kniebandersatz. Unfallchirurgie 11 (5): 242-246
27. Cusick JF, Myklebust J, Zyvoloski M (1982) Effects of vertebral column distraction in the monkey. J Neurosurg 57: 651-659
28. Dimitrijevic MR (1980) Neural control of locomotion in patients with spinal cord injury and effects of spinal cord stimulation. Transactions of 1st International Symposium on Spinal Cord Reconstruction, Las Vegas, Nevada, 7-10 Jan 1980
29. Dorian R (1985) Ist die operative Traktion der HWS noch zu befürworten? Z Orthop 123: 115-116
30. Dove J, Hsu LC, Yau ACMC (1980) The cervical spine after halopelvic traction. J Bone Joint Surg (Am) 62-3 (2): 158-161
31. Ducker TB (1976) Experimental injury of the spinal cord. In: Vinken PJ, Bruyn GW (eds) Handbook of clinical neurology, vol 25. North Holland, Amsterdam, pp 9-26
32. Feringa ER, Vahlsing HL, Woodard M (1984) Basal lamina at the site of spinal cord transection in the rat: an ultrastructural study. Neurosci Lett 51: 303-308
33. Frankel HL, Hancock DO, Hyslop G (1969) The value of postural reduction in the initial management of closed injuries of spine with paraplegia and tetraplegia. I. Paraplegia 7: 179-192
34. Gerfin SR, Botta MJ, Waters RC, Nickel VL (1986) Complications in the use of the halo fixation device. J Bone Joint Surg (Am) 68A: 320-325
35. Gledhill VX, Harrison BM, McDonald WI (1973) Demyelination and remyelination after acute spinal cord compression. Exp Neurol 38: 472-487
36. Glötzner FL, Netal R (1985) Conductivity in elastically stretched and relaxed spinal cord evaluated by somatosensory evoked potentials. In: Schramm J, Jones SJ (eds) Spinal cord monitoring. Springer, Berlin Heidelberg New York, pp 261-265
37. Goldsmith HS, Neil-Dwyer G, Barsoum L (1986) Omental transposition in the acute and chronically injured spinal cord. Paper presented at International Medical Society of Paraplegia meeting, Oslo, Norway, 26-28 June 1986
38. Guttmann L (1973) Spinal injuries: comprehensive management and research. Blackwell, Oxford
39. Illis LS, Sedgwick FM, Tallis RC (1980) Spinal cord stimulation in multiple sclerosis: clinical results. J Neurol Neurosurg Psychiatry 43: 1-14
40. Jellinger K (1976) Neuropathology of cord injuries. In: Vinken PJ, Bruyn GW (eds) Handbook of clinical neurology, vol 25. North Holland, Amsterdam, pp 43-121
41. Kaufmann HH, Harris JH, Spencer JA et al (1982) Danger of traction during radiography of cervical trauma. JAMA 247 (17): 2369
42. Kayan A, Earl CJ (1975) Compressive lesions of the optical nerves and chiasm. Pattern of recovery of vision following surgical treatment. Brain 98: 13-18

43. Key A, Retzius G (1875) Studien in der Anatomie des Nervensystems. Folio 166: 1, Norstedt, Stockholm
44. Louis R (1983) Surgery of the spine. Surgical and anatomy and operative approaches. Springer, Berlin Heidelberg New York
45. Mathur JG (1979) Indiscriminate use of traction in spinal injuries. Med J Aust 13: 1182
46. McDonald WI (1974) Remyelination in relation to clinical lesions of the central nervous system. Br Med Bull 30: 186-189
47. McMillan BS, Silver JR (1987) Extension injuries of the cervical spine resulting in tetraplegia. Injury 18: 224-233
48. McVeigh JF (1923) Experimental cord crushes, with a special reference to the mechanical factors involved and subsequent changes in areas of the cord affected. Arch Surg 7: 573-600
49. Morscher E, Jenny H, Olerud S, Suttor F (1986) Die vordere Verplattung der Halswirbelsäule mit dem Hohlschrauben-Plattensystem aus Titanium. Chirurg 57: 702-707
50. Olerud S, Karlström G (1979) Rigid internal fixation in fracture healing. In: McKibbin B (ed) Cardiff Recent advances in orthopaedics, 3rd edn. Churchill Livingstone, Edinburgh
51. Puchala E, Windle WF (1977) The possibility of structural and functional restitution after spinal cord injury: a review. Exp Neurol 55: 1-42
52. Roy-Camille R, Saillant G, Berteaux D, Serge M-A (1979) Early management of spinal cord injuries. In: McKibbin B (ed) Cardiff Recent advances in orthopaedics, 3rd edn. Churchill Livingstone, Edinburgh, pp 57-87
53. Ramon y Cajal S (1928) Degeneration and regeneration of the nervous system, vol 2. Translated and edited by RM May
54. Scher AT (1981) Overdistraction of cervical spinal injuries? S Afr Med J 59: 639-641
55. Sedgwick EM, El-Negami E, Frankel H (1980) Spinal cord potentials in traumatic paraplegia and tetraplegia. J Neurol Neurosurg Psychiatry 43: 823-830
56. Sedgwick EM (1982) Trial of spinal cord stimulation for rehabilitation of patients with spinal cord injury, International Spinal Research Trust Research Project
57. Shrosbree RD (1979) Neurological sequelae of reduction of fracture dislocations of the cervical spine. Paraplegia 17 (2): 212-221
58. Silver JR (1984) Injuries of the spine sustained in rugby. Br Med J 228: 37-43
59. Silver JR, Godfrey JJ (1986) Trampolining injuries of the spine. Injury 17: 117-124
60. Sonander H, Breig A, Dahlström A, Osawa M (1987) Effects on granulocytopoesis of pretreatment with slow-release vitamin B12 in prolonged exposure to 80% nitrous oxide in rats. Acta Anaesthesiol Scand (Submitted)
61. Taylor AR (1951) The mechanism of injury to the spinal cord in the neck without damage to the vertebral column. J Bone Joint Surg 338: 543-547
62. Thulin C-A (1981) Book review: Adverse mechanical tension in the central nervous system, Breig A. Acta Neurochirurgica 56 (1-2)
63. Toscano J (1986) Prevention of neurological deterioration before admission to a spinal cord injury unit. Paper read at International Medical Society of Paraplegia Meeting, Oslo, Norway, 26-28 June 1986
64. Transfeld EE, Simons EH (1982) Functional and pathological biomechanics of the spinal cord: an in vivo study. International Society for the Study of the Lumbar Spine (abstracts), Toronto, June 7
65. Turnbull IM, Breig A, Hassler O (1966) Blood supply of cervical spinal cord in man: a microangiographic cadaver study. J Neurosurg 24: 951-965
66. Wall PD (1986) Spinal cord injury. Criteria for judging research. A discussion document. August 1986. International Spinal Research Trust, Enfield, United Kingdom
67. White AA, Panjabi MM, Thomas CL (1977) The clinical biomechanics of kyphotic deformities. Clin Orthop Related Res 128: 8-17
68. White AA III, Panjabi MM (1978) Clinical biomechanics of the spine. Lippincott, Philadelphia
69. Wolman L (1965) The disturbance of circulation in traumatic paraplegia in acute and late stages: a pathological study. Paraplegia 2: 213-226

www.ingramcontent.com/pod-product-compliance
Ingram Content Group UK Ltd.
Pitfield, Milton Keynes, MK11 3LW, UK
UKHW051450290926
15471UKWH00008B/1119

* 9 7 8 3 5 4 0 5 0 4 1 4 6 *